CASE PROFILES IN
RESPIRATORY CARE

CASE PROFILES IN RESPIRATORY CARE

William A. French, MA, RRT
Director of Clinical Education
Respiratory Therapy Program
Lakeland Community College
Mentor, Ohio

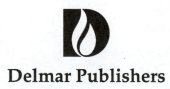

Delmar Publishers

I(T)P An International Thomson Publishing Company

Albany • Bonn • Boston • Cincinnati • Detroit • London • Madrid • Melbourne
Mexico City • New York • Pacific Grove • Paris • San Francisco • Singapore • Tokyo
Toronto • Washington

Cover Credit: Lauren Payne, Spiral Design Studio

Acquisitions Editor: Kimberly Davies
Developmental Editor: Debra Flis
Editorial Assistant: Donna Leto

Project Editor: Coreen Rogers
Production Coordinator: John Mickelbank
Art and Design Coordinator: Vincent S. Berger

Copyright © 1996
By Delmar Publishers
A Division of International Thomson Publishing Inc.

The ITP logo is a trademark under license

Printed in the United States of America

For more information, contact:

Delmar Publishers
3 Columbia Circle, Box 15015
Albany, New York 12212-5015

International Thomson Editores
Campos Eliseos 385, Piso 7
Col Polanco
11560 Mexico D F Mexico

International Thomson Publishing Europe
Berkshire House 168-173
High Holborn
London, WC1V7AA
England

International Thomson Publishing GmbH
Königswinterer Strasse 418
53227 Bonn
Germany

Thomas Nelson Australia
102 Dodds Street
South Melbourne, 3205
Victoria, Australia

International Thomson Publishing Asia
221 Henderson Road
#05-10 Henderson Building
Singapore 0315

Nelson Canada
1120 Birchmount Road
Scarborough, Ontario
Canada M1K 5G4

International Thomson Publishing - Japan
Hirakawacho Kyowa Building, 3F
2-2-1 Hirakawacho
Chiyoda-ku, Tokyo 102
Japan

1 2 3 4 5 6 7 8 9 10 XXX 01 00 99 98 97 96 95

Library of Congress Cataloging-in-Publication Data

French, William A.
　　Case profiles in respiratory care / William A. French.
　　　　p.　cm.
　　Includes bibliographical references.
　　ISBN 0-8273-6684-1 (alk. paper)
　　1. Respiratory therapy—Case studies.　I. Title.
　　[DNLM: 1. Respiratory Therapy—case studies.　2. Respiratory
Therapy—problems.　WB 18.2 F877c 1995]
RC735.I5F74　1996
615.8'36—dc20
DNLM/DLC
for Library of Congress　　　　　　　　　　　95-9196

CONTENTS

PREFACE

Purpose of the Book

The ability to solve patient related problems effectively and deal successfully with unique clinical situations in respiratory care is becoming increasingly critical. For recent graduates, this ability is tested thoroughly on the Clinical Simulation Exam administered by the National Board for Respiratory Care (NBRC). More importantly, however, this ability is needed every day on real patients in real world clinical settings, ranging from acute care hospitals to patients' homes. Quite often the clinician must quickly gather information and assess the situation, and then formulate and implement (or at least participate in the implementation of) an appropriate solution. In addition, many more hospitals are beginning to adopt therapist driven protocols in some form or another. Moreover, some respiratory care practitioners are currently, and many more will be, working from protocols in home care and skilled nursing facilities. Obviously, effective use of such protocols requires well developed critical thinking skills.

All of the indications strongly suggest that the respiratory care practitioners who will succeed in the future will be those who can gather relevant information, recognize specific cardiopulmonary problems, design and recommend an appropriate therapeutic course for each problem, and implement the therapy once prescribed. As is suggested by the relevant literature, this ability is one that is only developed through directed practice (Mishoe, 1993).

Unfortunately, as a student (or even as a clinician dedicated to a specific clinical setting) it is not always possible to experience all potential patient situations. It is possible, however, to integrate theory with actual practice and to expose students (and clinicians) to exercises that challenge and nurture their ability to work through complex clinical situations and to make appropriate decisions.

The purpose of this book is to present the learner with a series of patient situations and exercises of increasing complexity. At each level the learner will be asked to utilize the relevant information in order to make a decision about the patient's care. In the process the learner will be required to draw from relevant theory. This process of directed problem solving is based on the following premises:

1. Good decisions are made on the basis of relevant information.
2. Each patient encounter is truly unique.
3. Each patient problem may have more than one possible correct solution (e.g., a patient with COPD may benefit equally from a nasal cannula at 2 Lpm and an air entrainment mask at an FiO_2 of 0.28).

4. Solutions presented without a rational, well-structured explanation are not entirely correct. Thus, in this book solutions will be suggested for each patient situation. It will be left to the learner to supply alternative solutions and appropriate explanations in the case of disagreement. The author freely admits that there may be any number of appropriate therapeutic approaches to different patient situations; he only asks that these different approaches be defended.

How to Use the Book: Educators

This book was developed as a tool for teaching respiratory care students how to gather and use information to make informed decisions regarding the care of specific patients. Therefore, its primary use is in a generic respiratory care program. In that context it can be used in the following ways:

1. As an adjunct to classroom and laboratory discussions relative to a specific therapeutic modality or disease process (e.g., mechanical ventilation, COPD).
2. As a stand alone book of exercises for homework and out of class discussion.
3. As models for designing and implementing (in the classroom) procedure specific protocols.
4. As a catalyst for student problem creation (i.e., let the student create similar problems based on his/her own experience).
5. As models for laboratory simulations (especially the mechanical ventilation cases—these can be expanded and demonstrated on the appropriate equipment in the laboratory).

In addition to its use in the generic respiratory care program, this book can be used as a component of other health care programs (nursing in particular) and continuing education programs. In these contexts, the individual cases can be used as catalysts for the discussion of respiratory related issues. The fact that the answers provided are generally vague, and may not represent every clinician's viewpoint, make the cases all the more useful for stimulating discussion.

How to Use the Book: Students

As a student your patient related experience is necessarily limited. This book will expose you to patient situations that you might not have the opportunity to experience first hand.

However, the best way you can use this book is to learn to form your own conclusions and make convincing arguments for any therapeutic changes or programs you may want to implement. Discuss these cases with your instructors, fellow students, and active clinicians. Try to capture all possible therapeutic viewpoints and contingencies. When in doubt about an approach, attempt to simulate the patient situation in the laboratory. Only then will you be ready to assume the expanded role of the respiratory care practitioner.

Personal Note

I believe it is important to point out that each of the cases in this book is either real, drawn from personal experience (with names changed, of course), or a composite of several similar situations. The majority of the data is also real. Therefore, there should be no question about the reality of these situations even though some may not correspond completely with generic conventional wisdom (e.g., not all patients with COPD are CO_2 retainers).

On a more personal note, I have been a full time educator for nearly seventeen of my twenty-three years in respiratory therapy. For some of that time I did not engage in active practice. However, I found that my skills were eroding and that I did not have the proper perspective on the profession. Therefore, I sought out and found areas for active practice. Since making that decision nine years ago, I have worked (and continue to work) in acute care hospitals, a skilled nursing facility, home care, and an asthma camp. I believe this experience, apart from its obvious value to my teaching, has made me more sensitive to my students and to the profession.

ACKNOWLEDGMENTS

Throughout my adult life I have been truly blessed. I have been blessed with a family that has given me unconditional love and support. I have likewise been blessed with a profession that has provided me with continuous challenge, reward, and satisfaction. I do not believe that I shall ever grow tired of, or bored with, respiratory care.

I would like to first and foremost thank the thousands of patients that I have worked with over the years. Without them this project and our profession would obviously cease to exist. I would also like to thank the hundreds of students that I have had the privilege of teaching over the years. They have inspired me and taught me more than I could ever teach them.

Many individuals participated in some way in the completion of this project. Thank you to William Henry, RRT, who provided not only the neonatal cases in chapter five, but also constant inspiration and motivation. Thank you to the people at Delmar Publishers for pushing this project: First, Adrianne Williams and Jill Rembetski, then Kim Davies and her staff.

Finally, thank you to the individuals who reviewed the manuscript in its various stages: David Chang, EdD, RRT, Randy DeKler, RRT, Tim Op't Holt, EdD, RRT, Delmar Sieber, BS, RRT, and Sandra Gaviola, RRT.

CHAPTER ONE

PATIENT ASSESSMENT

INTRODUCTION

In this chapter, the learner is introduced to a series of patient situations. Each situation contains a brief physical description of the patient as he or she might be seen from the bedside. Each situation also contains physical assessment data that might be obtained from a standard pulmonary exam (i.e., observation, palpation, percussion, and auscultation). Basic cardiac data are also given. Each patient has some sort of fundamental cardiopulmonary disorder (e.g, COPD [Chronic Obstructive Pulmonary Disease], pneumothorax, consolidation/pneumonia, asthma, pulmonary edema, atelectasis, etc.). The nature of the cardiopulmonary problem should be relatively apparent from the assessment data given, and it is the task of the learner to determine what that problem is. The learner is *not diagnosing*, but rather recognizing a problem that may require some sort of respiratory therapy.

Some of the more advanced cases also contain basic lab data (e.g., arterial blood gas results, hematology values) to facilitate the recognition process. In all cases, the learner should have all the information she needs in order to successfully recognize the problem. In fact, in some cases, the learner may be given *more* information than she really needs. She should, however, look at all the information anyway.

——— **PREREQUISITE INFORMATION** ———

In order to successfully deal with each patient situation, the learner needs to have the following information:

1. Pulmonary physical assessment data:
   - breath sounds
   - chest movement and configuration
   - percussion/palpation
   - recognition of voiced sounds (e.g., egophony, bronchophony)
   - respiratory rate/rhythm/pattern

2. Basic cardiac assessment data:
   - pulse rate/force
   - blood pressure

3. Other physical assessment data:
   - temperature
   - mental status/affect
   - overall appearance (e.g., skin color, etc.)

4. Laboratory data:
   - arterial blood gas results (normal values only)
   - hematology (normal values only)

5. Basic awareness of the following cardiopulmonary problems:
   - chronic obstructive pulmonary disease (COPD)
   - asthma
   - consolidation/pneumonia
   - atelectasis
   - congestive heart failure/pulmonary edema
   - pneumothorax
   - pleural effusion

6. Basic medical terminology

The answers for each case appear in the appendix at the end of the text. More than one answer *may* be possible for each case (although not as likely as in chapters subsequent to Chapter One). As an additional exercise, the learner might want to suggest possible fundamental therapeutic approaches to each cardiopulmonary problem (e.g., the patient who has a pneumothorax will require a chest tube; a patient with hypoxemia will require oxygen, etc.)

PATIENT CASES

PATIENT 1 • Linda Loman

PATIENT: Linda Loman, a sixty-one-year-old female.
                    Admitted two days ago with a diagnosis of lung cancer.
                    Patient has now developed severe shortness of breath.
                    Patient is in a regular room with an IV.

PHYSICAL
FINDINGS: Decreased chest excursion on the left side; decreased
                    vocal fremitus in the left base; dull percussion note over
                    the left base; breath sounds are very decreased in the left
                    base, normal elsewhere.

• • •

Apparent Cardiopulmonary Problem:

Additional Useful Information:

Suggested Basic Treatment:

PATIENT 2 • Mary Malloy

PATIENT:

Mary Malloy, a seventy-year-old female.
Admitted yesterday with fever temperature of unknown origin.
Patient is apparently oriented but does not arouse easily; she is in a regular room with a peripheral IV and a foley catheter.

PHYSICAL FINDINGS:

Pulse 110, blood pressure (BP) 106/60, temperature 39°C, respirations 24, shallow with the left hemithorax expanding more than the right. The skin is warm and dry; she appears to be slightly cachectic. She has slightly increased vocal fremitus over the right middle lobe and dull percussion note over the right middle lobe; breath sounds are decreased throughout both lung fields with fine crackles over the right middle lobe.

• • •

Apparent Cardiopulmonary Problem:

Additional Useful Information:

Suggested Basic Treatment:

PATIENT 3 • J. C. Pierce

PATIENT:

J. C. Pierce, a fifty-year-old male.
Seen in the emergency department for shortness of
breath of sudden onset.
Patient is alert and oriented, but very anxious.

**PHYSICAL
FINDINGS:**

Pulse 120, BP 160/90, temperature 37.2°C, respirations
25, shallow and slightly labored. Chest expansion is
decreased bilaterally; slightly decreased vocal fremitus
throughout; dull percussion note throughout; breath
sounds are decreased bilaterally with course crackles on
inspiration throughout. Patient's skin is warm and
moist; lips and nailbeds are slightly cyanotic.

• • •

Apparent Cardiopulmonary Problem:

Additional Useful Information:

Suggested Basic Treatment:

PATIENT 4 • Jake McCandles

PATIENT:
Jake McCandles, a forty-five-year-old male.
Admitted two days ago with a diagnosis of
pneumonia.
Patient is responsive only to painful stimuli. Patient is
in a monitored bed, has a central IV line and a foley
catheter.

PHYSICAL
FINDINGS:
Pulse 94, BP 148/84, temperature 38.2°C, respirations
22, shallow. Chest expansion is decreased on the right
side; percussion note is dull over the right side. Breath
sounds are decreased throughout both lungs, slightly
bronchial over the right side, especially the base.
Patient's skin is warm and dry.

• • •

Apparent Cardiopulmonary Problem:

Additional Useful Information:

Suggested Basic Treatment:

—————— **PATIENT 5** • **Alex Dwyer** ——————

PATIENT:

Alex Dwyer, a fifty-four-year-old male.
Admitted this morning with a chief complaint of shortness of breath.
Patient is alert and oriented, but very anxious. Patient is in a regular room with a peripheral IV.

PHYSICAL
FINDINGS:

Pulse 106, BP 136/82, temperature 37.4°C, respirations 24, slightly labored with use of accessory muscles. Chest excursion is decreased bilaterally; slightly decreased vocal fremitus, slightly hyperresonant percussion note. Breath sounds are decreased with wheezing superimposed over a prolonged expiratory phase throughout both lungs. Patient has difficulty completing a sentence.

• • •

Apparent Cardiopulmonary Problem:

Additional Useful Information:

Suggested Basic Treatment:

—————— **PATIENT 6** • Katherine McClintock ——————

PATIENT:

Katherine McClintock, a fifty-four-year-old female. Admitted through the emergency department with chest trauma from an automobile accident. Patient is anxious and confused; she has a peripheral IV and is in the intensive care unit.

PHYSICAL
FINDINGS:

Pulse 132, BP 94/40, temperature 36.2°C, respirations 28, very shallow. Chest excursion is decreased on the left side; percussion note is hyperresonant over the left side, slightly dull over the right side. Breath sounds are decreased on the right side, absent on the left side.

• • •

Apparent Cardiopulmonary Problem:

Additional Useful Information:

Suggested Basic Treatment:

──────── **PATIENT 7** • **Fenton Hardy** ────────

PATIENT:

Fenton Hardy, an eighty-year-old male.
Admitted last night from a nursing home with a diagnosis of pneumonia.
Patient is unresponsive. Patient has a peripheral IV and a central line; he has a feeding tube in place and a foley catheter.

PHYSICAL FINDINGS:

Pulse 110, regular, BP 152/96, temperature 39°C, respirations 24, shallow and slightly labored. The left hemithorax is expanding more than the right; percussion note is dull over right base. Breath sounds are decreased in both bases with rhonchi on expiration, and fine crackles on inspiration in the right base.

LAB DATA:

pH 7.52, $PaCO_2$ 26, HCO_3- 21, PaO_2 53, SaO_2 91%, FiO_2 0.21, hemoglobin (Hgb) 11.4, hematocrit 38, white blood cell count (WBC) 12,200.

• • •

Apparent Cardiopulmonary Problem:

Additional Useful Information:

Suggested Basic Treatment:

—————— **PATIENT 8** • **Chet Morton** ——————

PATIENT: Chet Morton, a forty-two-year-old male.
Patient was admitted yesterday with an exacerbation of COPD.
Patient is alert and oriented. He has a peripheral IV and is in a regular room.

PHYSICAL
FINDINGS: Pulse 98, regular, BP 146/88, temperature 38.2°C, respirations 22, shallow and labored with use of accessory muscles. Chest excursion is decreased bilaterally; vocal fremitus and percussion notes are mostly normal throughout both lung fields. Breath sounds are very decreased, especially in the bases; some rhonchi are heard on exhalation. Patient's lips and nail beds are slightly cyanotic.

LAB DATA: pH 7.36, $PaCO_2$ 54, HCO_3- 30, PaO_2 58, SaO_2 88%, FiO_2 nasal cannula at 2 Lpm; Hgb 17.4, hematocrit 48, WBC 11,300.

• • •

Apparent Cardiopulmonary Problem:

Additional Useful Information:

Suggested Basic Treatment:

PATIENT 9 • Wilma Wagg

PATIENT: Wilma Wagg, a sixty-five-year-old female.
Admitted this morning with an apparent exacerbation of COPD.
Patient is alert and oriented. She is in a regular room with a peripheral IV.

PHYSICAL FINDINGS: Pulse 110, regular, BP 138/90, temperature 38°C, respirations 24, slightly labored. Chest excursion is decreased throughout; vocal fremitus is slightly decreased; percussion note is slightly hyperresonant throughout. Breath sounds are very decreased, especially in bases, expiratory phase is prolonged. Patient is sitting up in bed, leaning on the bedside table. She is exhaling through pursed lips.

LAB DATA: pH 7.44, $PaCO_2$ 32, HCO_3- 23, PaO_2 50, SaO_2 87%, FiO_2 nasal cannula 1 Lpm; Hgb 12.6, hematocrit 42, WBC 10,200.

• • •

Apparent Cardiopulmonary Problem:

Additional Useful Information:

Suggested Basic Treatment:

PATIENT 10 • Trisha Foder

PATIENT:
Trisha Foder, a thirty-year-old female.
Admitted through the emergency department with shortness of breath of relatively rapid onset.
Patient is alert and oriented, but very anxious. She is in a regular room on nasal oxygen at 4 Lpm.

PHYSICAL
FINDINGS:
Pulse 134, regular, BP 156/84, temperature 37.4°C, respirations 30, very labored. Chest expansion is decreased bilaterally; vocal fremitus is normal, percussion note is slightly hyperresonant. Breath sounds are very decreased with a prolonged expiratory phase. Patient is sitting up in bed.

LAB DATA:
pH 7.52, $PaCO_2$ 28, HCO_3- 24, PaO_2 76, SaO_2 96%, Hgb 13.2, hematocrit 43, WBC 11,300.

• • •

Apparent Cardiopulmonary Problem:

Additional Useful Information:

Suggested Basic Treatment:

CHAPTER TWO

INTERPRETING ORDERS

INTRODUCTION

In the last chapter, the learner was given basic physical assessment data about the patient and was asked to determine the cardiopulmonary problem. He was also asked to suggest basic therapeutic modalities. In this chapter, the learner is given a patient scenario and orders for therapy. The learner's task is to examine these orders and determine whether or not they are appropriate for the particular patient. In determining this appropriateness, the learner will ask two questions:

1) "Are the orders *technically correct*?" (that is, do the orders conform to generally accepted respiratory therapy practice?)
2) "If the orders are technically correct, are they appropriate for the patient?" (that is, will the therapy, if properly implemented, very likely correct the patient's cardiopulmonary problems *without causing undue harm in the process*?)

In some cases, the learner may not agree completely with the orders, but not find them particularly harmful . In such cases, he must ask himself if he would call the physician in the middle of the night to argue for change, or if he would implement the orders as they are and then assess their effectiveness. If the learner decides that orders must be changed, he must: 1) state specifically why the orders need to be changed and 2) recommend detailed alternatives along with rationale.

Since respiratory care practitioners (RCPs) must act (in some form) according to physician's orders, this chapter is particularly crucial, especially in reinforcing skills that will enable RCPs to interact with physicians in determining the best therapeutic course for their patients. As in other chapters in this book, many answers may be possible for some cases. However, in cases where there is significant disagreement between the book's answer and the learner, the learner must be prepared to defend his answer with sound reasoning.

All of the cases in this chapter revolve around basic cardiopulmonary situations. If the learner believes that the patient would benefit from some sort of assisted ventilation, he need only say so; he is not expected to make specific recommendations as to type of assisted ventilation.

—— PREREQUISITE INFORMATION ——

In order to successfully deal with the cases in this chapter, the learner must have the following information:

1. All of the information detailed in chapter one.
2. Type and specifications for oxygen delivery devices.
3. Indications and hazards for oxygen therapy.
4. Types and specifications for aerosol delivery devices.
5. Indications and hazards for aerosol therapy.
6. Indications, hazards, and dosing information for all currently available inhaled medications (including those available only by metered dose inhaler).
7. Indications and hazards of intermittent positive pressure breathing (IPPB).
8. Indications for incentive spirometry.
9. Indications for breathing retraining exercises (diaphragmatic and pursed lip breathing).
10. Indications and hazards for chest physical therapy (chest percussion, postural drainage, and vibration).
11. Basic blood gas interpretation, including oxygenation.
12. Signs and symptoms of secretion retention.

Some of the cases are marked with a D. These have some additional considerations that should be discussed (i.e., problems that complicate therapy that are unique to that patient).

PATIENT CASES

PATIENT 1 • I. M. Quick

PATIENT:
I. M. Quick, a forty-nine-year-old male.
Admitted with an exacerbation of COPD.
Patient is alert but slightly confused.

PHYSICAL
FINDINGS:
Pulse 120, regular, BP 136/90, temperature 38°C, respirations 24, slightly labored. Breath sounds are decreased in bases with prolonged expiratory phase. Loose, nonproductive cough. Patient has an IV and is in a regular room.

LAB DATA:
pH 7.32, $PaCO_2$ 59, HCO_3- 32, PaO_2 50, SaO_2 84%, FiO_2 0.21, WBC 11,200, Hgb 13.3, hematocrit 44.

ORDER:
O_2 via 0.28 Venturi (air entrainment) mask.

• • •

Would you implement this order as it is written? What would you recommend in its place? Would you add or delete anything from this order?

——————— **PATIENT 2** • Adolph Petroni ———————

PATIENT:

Adolph Petroni, a seventy-two-year-old male. Admitted this morning through the emergency department for shortness of breath secondary to COPD. Patient is alert and oriented, and is in a regular room.

PHYSICAL
FINDINGS:

Pulse 120, regular, BP 140/80, temperature 38.2°C, respirations 24, labored. Breath sounds decreased throughout with rhonchi superimposed over a prolonged expiratory phase. Patient has a productive cough with thick yellow sputum.

LAB DATA:

pH 7.44, $PaCO_2$ 58, HCO_3^- 38, PaO_2 50, SaO_2 83%, FiO_2 0.21, WBC 9,800, Hgb 16.9, hematocrit 49.

ORDER:

Oxygen via nasal cannula at 6 Lpm.

• • •

Would you implement this order as it is written? What would you recommend in its place? Would you add or delete anything from this order?

PATIENT 3 • Mary Pusche

PATIENT:
Mary Pusche, a seventy-year-old female. Admitted last night with a diagnosis of lung cancer. Patient is alert and oriented. She is on the oncology unit and is receiving chemotherapy.

PHYSICAL
FINDINGS:
Pulse 132, regular, BP 96/40, temperature 37.6°C, respirations 32, shallow. Breath sounds are decreased throughout with fine crackles on inspiration. Chest expansion is decreased in both bases.

LAB DATA:
pH 7.52, $PaCO_2$ 26, HCO_3- 21, PaO_2 45, SaO_2 86%, FiO_2 0.21, WBC 3,800, Hgb 8.6, hematocrit 28.

ORDER:
Oxygen via simple mask at 3 Lpm.

• • •

Would you implement this order as it is written? What would you recommend in its place? Would you add or delete anything from this order?

——————— **PATIENT 4** • **Philip Folkstone** ———————

PATIENT: Philip Folkstone, a thirty-six-year old male.
                       Admitted through the emergency department with
                       pulmonary edema secondary to congestive heart
                       failure. Patient is alert but anxious; he is on a cardiac
                       monitor in the coronary care unit.

PHYSICAL
FINDINGS: Pulse 140, thready, BP 106/60, temperature 36.9°C,
                       respirations 34, shallow and labored. Breath sounds
                       decreased throughout with coarse crackles on
                       inspiration; chest expansion is decreased. Patient is
                       sitting up in bed and is diaphoretic.

LAB DATA: pH 7.50, $PaCO_2$ 28, HCO_3^- 22, PaO_2 48, SaO_2 85%, FiO_2
                       nasal cannula at 2 Lpm. No other blood work done.

ORDER: Increase oxygen to 4 Lpm.

• • •

Would you implement this order as it is written? What would you recommend in
its place? Would you add or delete anything from this order?

PATIENT 5 • Bronco Lane

PATIENT:
Bronco Lane, a fifty-nine-year-old male.
Admitted this morning with acute dyspnea secondary to pulmonary fibrosis. Patient is alert and oriented; he is in a regular room and has an IV.

PHYSICAL
FINDINGS:
Pulse 120, regular, BP 146/90, temperature 39°C, respirations 28, shallow, labored. Breath sounds are decreased throughout with fine crackles on inspiration, chest expansion is decreased in both bases. The patient is not coughing.

LAB DATA:
pH 7.52, $PaCO_2$ 30, HCO_3- 24, PaO_2 42, SaO_2 80%, FiO_2 0.21, Hgb 10.2, WBC 9,400.

ORDER:
Oxygen via nasal catheter at 2 Lpm.

• • •

Would you implement this order as it is written? What would you recommend in its place? Would you add or delete anything from this order?

───────── **PATIENT 6 • Brewster Baker** ─────────

PATIENT:
Brewster Baker, a forty-five-year-old male.
Admitted through the emergency department with a
probable myocardial infarction (pending outcome of
cardiac enzymes). Patient is alert and very anxious, he
is in the coronary unit on a monitor.

PHYSICAL
FINDINGS:
Pulse 146, irregular, BP 166/102, temperature 37.2°C,
respirations 26, slightly labored. Breath sounds
normal, chest expansion mostly normal. No coughing.
Patient is sitting in semi-Fowlers position and is
slightly diaphoretic.

LAB DATA:
pH 7.50, $PaCO_2$ 29, HCO_3- 23, PaO_2 72, SaO_2 96%, FiO_2
0.21, other blood work pending.

ORDER:
Oxygen via simple mask at 5 Lpm.

• • •

Would you implement this order as it is written? What would you recommend in
its place? Would you add or delete anything from this order?

——————— **PATIENT 7** • **Laurie Cable** ———————

PATIENT: Laurie Cable, a twenty-six-year-old female.
Admitted to the emergency room with acute onset of
shortness of breath. Patient is alert and somewhat
anxious, she is seen in the emergency room.

PHYSICAL
FINDINGS: Pulse 136, regular, BP 146/88, temperature 38°C,
respirations 26, shallow and labored. Breath sounds
decreased throughout with wheezing superimposed
over a prolonged expiratory phase. Patient has a dry,
nonproductive cough and nasal congestion.

LAB DATA: SpO_2 (pulse oximeter) 92% on room air.

ORDER: Oxygen via nasal cannula at 6 Lpm.

• • •

Would you implement this order as it is written? What would you recommend in
its place? Would you add or delete anything from this order?

———— **PATIENT 8** • Marion Ravenwood ————

PATIENT: Marion Ravenwood, a thirty-six-year-old female. Admitted two days ago with a prolapsed uterus. Had a hysterectomy yesterday. Patient is alert and oriented, she is in a regular room on the surgical floor, she has an IV.

PHYSICAL
FINDINGS: Pulse 110, regular, BP 152/86, temperature 38.6°C, respirations 26, shallow. Breath sounds decreased, especially in the bases, fine crackles in the bases. Patient has a weak, nonproductive cough.

LAB DATA: SpO_2 (pulse oximeter) 93%, Hgb 12.4, WBC 12,200.

ORDER: Oxygen via 35% Venturi (air entrainment) mask.

• • •

Would you implement this order as it is written? What would you recommend in its place? Would you add or delete anything from this order?

PATIENT 9 • Julio Delgado

PATIENT: Julio Delgado, a sixty-four-year-old male. Admitted last night with an acute exacerbation of chronic bronchiectasis. Patient is alert but anxious, he is in a regular room and has an IV.

PHYSICAL
FINDINGS: Pulse 112, regular, BP 152/90, temperature 38.4°C, respirations 24, shallow, slightly labored. Breath sounds decreased with rhonchi on exhalation throughout both lungs. Patient has a weak productive cough with moderate amounts of thick, yellowish sputum. Patient is sitting up in bed.

LAB DATA: pH 7.46, $PaCO_2$ 38, HCO_3- 25, PaO_2 54, SaO_2 90%, FiO_2 0.21, Hgb 17.4, WBC 13,200.

ORDER: Oxygen via nasal cannula at 4 Lpm.

• • •

Would you implement this order as it is written? What would you recommend in its place? Would you add or delete anything from this order?

PATIENT 10 • Wilma Dearing

PATIENT: Wilma Dearing, a fifty-year-old female.
                            Admitted this afternoon with acute shortness of breath
                            secondary to COPD. Patient is alert and oriented; she
                            is in a regular room and has an IV.

PHYSICAL
FINDINGS: Pulse 102, regular, BP 138/80, temperature 38.3°C,
                            respirations 22, slightly labored. Breath sounds
                            decreased throughout with rhonchi on exhalation in
                            bases. Patient has occasional productive cough of
                            thick, greenish sputum. Patient is sitting up in bed.

LAB DATA: pH 7.32, $PaCO_2$ 58, HCO_3- 30, PaO_2 62, SaO_2 90%, FiO_2
                            via nasal cannula at 3 Lpm, Hgb 16.2, WBC 11,200.

ORDER: Increase oxygen to 60% by aerosol mask.

• • •

Would you implement this order as it is written? What would you recommend in
its place? Would you add or delete anything from this order?

———— **PATIENT 11** • Gracie Kleidsdale ————

PATIENT: Gracie Kleidsdale, an eighty-year-old female.
                    Admitted yesterday from a nursing home for
                    dehydration and confusion. Patient is arousable and
                    confused. She is in a regular room with an IV.

PHYSICAL
FINDINGS: Pulse 86, thready, BP 84/50, temperature 38.4°C,
                    respirations 28, shallow. Breath sounds very
                    decreased, with scattered rhonchi. Chest expansion
                    decreased, especially in the bases. Occasional weak,
                    dry nonproductive cough. Patient is thin with warm,
                    dry skin.

LAB DATA: pH 7.46, $PaCO_2$ 32, HCO_3- 25, PaO_2 49, SaO_2 82%, FiO_2
                    0.21, Hgb 10.2, WBC 11,200.

ORDER: Incentive spirometry Q. 2h.

• • •

Would you implement this order as it is written? What would you recommend in
its place? Would you add or delete anything from this order?

PATIENT 12 • Gene Crisby

PATIENT:	Gene Crisby, a forty-four-year-old male. Admitted this afternoon with what appears to be a myasthenic crisis (patient has a history of myasthenia gravis). Patient is alert and oriented. He is in the intensive care unit.
PHYSICAL FINDINGS:	Pulse 86, regular, BP 128/80, temperature 37°C, respirations 24, shallow. Breath sounds decreased throughout, chest expansion decreased in the bases. Patient is not coughing. He is in the semi-Fowlers position in bed and complains of some extremity weakness and some dysphagia.
LAB DATA:	SpO_2 94% on room air.
ORDERS:	IPPB with 3cc normal saline at a maximum pressure of 15 cm H_2O for ten minutes Q. 2h.

• • •

Would you implement this order as it is written? What would you recommend in its place? Would you add or delete anything from this order?

PATIENT 13 • Winnie Kirkwood

PATIENT: Winnie Kirkwood, a seventy-six-year-old female. Admitted this morning with shortness of breath progressing over the last 24 hours. Patient has a history of COPD. Patient is alert and possibly confused. She is in a regular room.

PHYSICAL
FINDINGS: Pulse 108, regular, BP 102/70, temperature 38.4°C, respirations 22, shallow. Breath sounds decreased with rhonchi in bases. Patient has an occasional cough which appears to be productive—patient is swallowing mucous. The patient is in semi-Fowler's position, she is slightly overweight.

LAB DATA: pH 7.37, $PaCO_2$ 60, HCO_3- 34, PaO_2 46, SaO_2 78%, FiO_2 nasal cannula at 1 Lpm, Hgb 15.8, WBC 13,100.

ORDERS: Increase oxygen to 5 Lpm.
Administer 2 puffs ventolin via metered dose inhaler (MDI) Q. 4h.

• • •

Would you implement this order as it is written? What would you recommend in its place? Would you add or delete anything from this order?

─────────── **PATIENT 14 • Kip Kiester** ───────────

PATIENT: Kip Kiester, a fifty-two-year-old male.
                      Patient had a colon resection two days ago.
                      Patient is alert and oriented. He is in a regular room on
                      the surgical floor. Patient has a thirty pack-year
                      smoking history.

PHYSICAL
FINDINGS: Pulse 110, regular, BP 158/90, temperature 38.8°C,
                      respirations 24, shallow. Breath sounds are decreased
                      with rhonchi on exhalation throughout. Chest
                      expansion is decreased in the bases. Patient has
                      occasional weak, nonproductive cough. Skin is warm
                      and moist.

LAB DATA: SpO_2 94% on room air.

ORDERS: Incentive spirometry Q. 2h.
                      Administer 0.5cc isoetharine in 2.5cc normal saline via
                      aerosol q.i.d.

• • •

Would you implement this order as it is written? What would you recommend in
its place? Would you add or delete anything from this order?

—————— **PATIENT 15** • Jonathan Harker ——————

PATIENT:
Jonathan Harker, a seventy-year-old male.
Admitted this morning with an exacerbation of
ulcerative colitis. Patient has a long history of COPD.
Patient is alert and oriented. He is in a regular room
and has an IV.

PHYSICAL
FINDINGS:
Pulse 98, regular, BP 134/92, temperature 37.6°C,
respirations 22. Breath sounds clear in apices, scattered
rhonchi in the bases, occasional productive cough of
white sputum. Patient is resting comfortably in bed.

LAB DATA:
SpO_2 92% on 2 Lpm via nasal cannula, Hgb 12.8, WBC
12,300.

ORDERS:
Increase oxygen to 4 Lpm.
0.5cc isoetharine in 2.5cc normal saline via aerosol
Q. 4h.

• • •

Would you implement this order as it is written? What would you recommend in
its place? Would you add or delete anything from this order?

PATIENT 16 • Mina Seward

PATIENT: Mina Seward, a sixty-year-old female.
Admitted last night from a nursing home with
increasing shortness of breath and increased
temperature. Patient is minimally responsive. She is in
a regular room with an IV.

PHYSICAL
FINDINGS: Pulse 104, thready, BP 96/42, temperature 38.8°C,
respirations 30, shallow. Breath sounds are decreased
throughout with rhonchi on exhalation. Patient has
occasional weak, nonproductive cough. Patient's skin
is warm and dry.

LAB DATA: pH 7.52, $PaCO_2$ 28, HCO_3- 23, PaO_2 44, SaO_2 83%, FiO_2
0.21, Hgb 10.2, WBC 11,200.

ORDERS: Oral intubation, place on 60% oxygen via aerosol T-
tube to an ET (endotracheal) tube.

• • •

Would you implement this order as it is written? What would you recommend in
its place? Would you add or delete anything from this order?

——————   **PATIENT 17** • **Adam Troy**   ——————

PATIENT: Adam Troy, a seventy-five-year-old male.
                  Admitted this morning with an exacerbation COPD.
                  Patient is alert and oriented. He is in a regular room
                  with an IV.

PHYSICAL
FINDINGS: Pulse 96, regular, BP 134/82, temperature 38.3°C,
                  respirations 24, shallow. Breath sounds decreased in
                  the bases with rhonchi on exhalation throughout,
                  occasional productive cough of thick greenish sputum.
                  Patient is sitting up in bed.

LAB DATA: pH 7.42, $PaCO_2$ 38, HCO_3- 24, PaO_2 56, SaO_2 91%, FiO_2
                  0.21, Hgb 14.6, WBC 13,400.

ORDERS: Oxygen via nasal cannula at 2 Lpm.
                  0.3cc metaproterenol in 2.1cc normal saline Q. 4h.

• • •

Would you implement this order as it is written? What would you recommend in its place? Would you add or delete anything from this order?

PATIENT 18 • Duke Lukela

PATIENT:

Duke Lukela, a forty-two-year-old male. Admitted this afternoon with an exacerbation of silicosis. Patient is alert and oriented. He is in a regular room with an IV in place.

PHYSICAL FINDINGS:

Pulse 96, regular, BP 134/90, temperature 38°C, respirations 26, shallow. Breath sounds are very decreased throughout; chest expansion is very decreased throughout. Patient is not coughing.

LAB DATA:

pH 7.42, $PaCO_2$ 30, HCO_3- 19, PaO_2 58, SaO_2 82%, FiO_2 nasal cannula at 2 Lpm, Hgb 16.4, WBC 10,600.

ORDERS:

Increase oxygen to 5 Lpm.
Atrovent 2 puffs Q. 6h.

• • •

Would you implement this order as it is written? What would you recommend in its place? Would you add or delete anything to this order?

────── **PATIENT 19** • Philip Hogan ──────

PATIENT:
Philip Hogan, a sixty-year-old male.
He had a large bowel resection yesterday.
Patient is alert and oriented. He is on the surgical floor and has an IV in place.

PHYSICAL
FINDINGS:
Pulse 110, regular, BP 146/82, temperature 38.4°C, respirations 26, shallow. Breath sounds decreased with fine crackles in the right base, chest expansion is decreased on both sides, less on the right. Patient has occasional weak, nonproductive cough.

LAB DATA:
SpO_2 90% on room air.

ORDERS:
Oxygen at 2 Lpm via nasal cannula.
IPPB with 0.3cc metaproterenol in 2.1cc normal saline q.i.d.

• • •

Would you implement this order as it is written? What would you recommend in its place? Would you add or delete anything from this order?

————————— **PATIENT 20 • Ann Fan** —————————

PATIENT:

Ann Fan, a fifty-two-year-old female.
Admitted through the emergency department with an
exacerbation of emphysema. Patient is oriented but
somewhat lethargic.

PHYSICAL
FINDINGS:

Pulse 88, regular, BP 110/70, temperature 38.2°C,
respirations 24, shallow. Breath sounds are very
decreased throughout. Chest expansion is decreased,
especially in the bases. Patient has occasional weak,
nonproductive cough. Patient is in semi-Fowler's
position and has warm, dry skin.

LAB DATA:

pH 7.48, $PaCO_2$ 34, HCO_3- 23, PaO_2 55, SaO_2 91%, FiO_2
nasal cannula at 1 Lpm, Hgb 13.8, WBC 9,800.

ORDERS:

Increase oxygen to 3 Lpm.
IPPB with 0.5cc albuterol in 2cc 20% mucomyst Q. 4h.

• • •

Would you implement this order as it is written? What would you recommend in
its place? Would you add or delete anything from this order?

PATIENT 21 • Wilbur Post

PATIENT:

Wilbur Post, a fifty-two-year-old male.
Admitted through the emergency department with acute onset of shortness of breath. Patient has a long history of congestive heart failure. Patient is alert and very anxious. He is on an emergency room cart.

PHYSICAL
FINDINGS:

Pulse 132, bounding, BP 178/96, temperature 37.2°C, respirations 30, shallow and labored. Breath sounds decreased throughout with coarse crackles in all fields. The patient is not coughing. His skin is warm and moist. He is sitting up in bed in apparent respiratory distress.

LAB DATA:

pH 7.39, $PaCO_2$ 45, HCO_3- 26, PaO_2 41, SaO_2 76%, FiO_2 0.21.

ORDERS:

Oxygen via nasal cannula at 6 Lpm.
0.5cc albuterol in 2.5cc normal saline stat.

• • •

Would you implement this order as it is written? What would you recommend in its place? Would you add or delete anything from this order?

——————— **PATIENT 22 • Peter Valdez** ———————

PATIENT: Peter Valdez, a forty-three-year-old male.
Admitted last night with a stab wound to the left
thorax, wound was repaired in surgery.
Patient is alert and somewhat belligerent, he is in the
intensive care unit and has a chest tube in the left
hemithorax.

PHYSICAL
FINDINGS: Pulse 120, regular, BP 148/90, temperature 38°C,
respirations 32, shallow. Breath sounds are very
decreased over the left base; chest expansion is
decreased on the left side. The patient is not coughing.
The chest tube is draining serosanguineous fluid.

LAB DATA: pH 7.48, $PaCO_2$ 26, HCO_3- 19, PaO_2 66, SaO_2 94%, FiO_2
0.35 (via air entrainment mask), Hgb 11.4, WBC 11,200.

ORDERS: Increase oxygen to 50%.
IPPB with 0.5cc albuterol in 2.5cc normal saline Q. 4h.

• • •

Would you implement this order as it is written? What would you recommend in
its place? Would you add or delete anything from this order?

PATIENT 23 • Helena Troy

PATIENT:

Helena Troy, a thirty-year-old female.
Admitted last night for acute shortness of breath; patient has a long history of asthma.
Patient is alert and oriented, she is in a regular room with an IV.

PHYSICAL FINDINGS:

Pulse 106, regular, BP 146/84, temperature 37.8°C, respirations 26, shallow, slightly labored. Breath sounds decreased with wheezing superimposed over a prolonged expiratory phase in all fields. The patient has an occasional nonproductive cough. She is sitting up in bed.

LAB DATA:

pH 7.49, $PaCO_2$ 30, HCO_3- 23, PaO_2 76, SaO_2 96%, FiO_2 nasal cannula 2 Lpm, Hgb 14.8, WBC 9,800, peak flow 210 Lpm.

ORDERS:

Increase oxygen to 4 Lpm.
Ventolin 2 puffs Q. 4h. via metered dose inhaler.
Atrovent 2 puffs Q. 6h. via metered dose inhaler.

• • •

Would you implement this order as it is written? What would you recommend in its place? Would you add or delete anything from this order?

——— **PATIENT 24 (D)** • **Missy Kosnowski** ———

PATIENT:
Missy Kosnowski, a fifteen-year-old female.
Admitted this morning for acute exacerbation of cystic fibrosis.
Patient is alert but is severely retarded (able to function at the five to six year old level). This is her third admission in the past twelve months for the same problem.

PHYSICAL
FINDINGS:
Pulse 106, regular, BP 114/70, temperature 38.2°C, respirations 32, shallow. Breath sounds are very decreased with some rhonchi heard in the apices, chest expansion is decreased on both sides. The patient has an occasional cough, sometimes productive of thick, tenacious yellowish sputum.

LAB DATA:
SpO_2 89% on oxygen at 2 Lpm via nasal cannula.

ORDERS:
0.5cc isoetharine in 2cc 10% mucomyst Q. 4h.

• • •

Would you implement this order as it is written? What would you recommend in its place? Would you add or delete anything from this order?

PATIENT 25 (D) · Judy Dooby

PATIENT:
Judy Dooby, an eight-year-old female.
Admitted yesterday following an auto accident in which she suffered compound fractures of the right and left femurs, and left patella, she also suffered some contusions on the arms and face.
Patient is alert and oriented, she is in traction on the pediatric floor.

PHYSICAL FINDINGS:
Pulse 98, regular, BP 98/60, temperature 38.8°C, respirations 26, shallow. Breath sounds very decreased in bases, chest expansion is decreased on both sides. The patient has an occasional weak, nonproductive cough.

LAB DATA:
SpO_2 94% on room air.

ORDERS:
Oxygen via nasal cannula at 2 Lpm.
Incentive spirometry Q. 2h.

• • •

Would you implement this order as it is written? What would you recommend in its place? Would you add or delete anything from this order?

CHAPTER THREE

RECOMMENDING TREATMENT

─── INTRODUCTION ───

In the last chapter, the learner was given a patient scenario and a prescription for treatment. The learner was then asked to determine if that prescription was appropriate for the patient. If the learner determined that the order was inappropriate, he or she was to state why and give specific recommendations for an alternative. That type of exercise is consistent with common practice since respiratory care still needs to be prescribed by a physician. However, in some health care facilities respiratory care practitioners are given the freedom to make specific therapeutic decisions on the basis of established protocols (therapist driven protocols). In still other facilities, physicians are asking for specific recommendations.

The purpose of the exercises in this chapter is to give the learner the opportunity to recommend therapy based on a patient scenario without first reacting to a physician order. The learner may make recommendations based on established protocols used in affiliate health care facilities or based on instructor generated criteria. The answers supplied are correspondingly vague—it is not the purpose of this book to promote any *specific* set of protocols or treatment philosophy.

Specifically, in dealing with each patient scenario, the learner is asked two questions:

1) "What specific respiratory related therapeutic modalities do you recommend at this time?"

2) "What is your rationale for these specific modalities?" (The answer should be in the form of orders as they would appear in a chart.)

In recommending treatment, the learner may select any non-invasive therapeutic modality currently in use (including continuous positive air pressure (CPAP) and the administration of any inhalation drug, either by MDI (metered dose inhaler) or small volume nebulizer.

—— PREREQUISITE INFORMATION ——

In order to successfully deal with the cases in this chapter, the learner must have the following information:

1. All of the information detailed in chapter one.
2. Type and specifications for oxygen delivery devices.
3. Indications and hazards for oxygen therapy.
4. Types and specifications for aerosol delivery devices.
5. Indications and hazards for aerosol therapy.
6. Indications, hazards, and dosing information for all currently available inhaled medications (including those available only by metered dose inhaler).
7. Indications and hazards of intermittent positive pressure breathing (IPPB).
8. Indications for incentive spirometry.
9. Indications for breathing retraining exercises (diaphragmatic and pursed lip breathing).
10. Indications and hazards for chest physical therapy (chest percussion, postural drainage, and vibration).
11. Basic blood gas interpretation, including oxygenation.
12. Signs and symptoms of secretion retention.

Some of the cases are marked with a D. These have some additional considerations that should be discussed (i.e., problems that complicate therapy that are unique to that patient).

PATIENT CASES

PATIENT 1 • Katherine Didd

PATIENT:

Katherine Didd, a thirty-seven-year-old female was seen in the emergency department with multiple trauma from a car accident. Patient is sitting up on the cart; she is alert and oriented. She appears to have some facial wounds. She has an IV running in the right hand.

PHYSICAL
FINDINGS:

Pulse 142, regular, BP 152/78, temperature 37.4°C, respirations 28, shallow, slightly labored. The right hemithorax appears to be expanding more than the left. Breath sounds are decreased throughout, absent on the left, percussion note is dull over the left base.

LAB DATA:

SpO_2 88% on a nasal cannula running at 6 Lpm; all other lab work pending.

• • •

The attending physician asks you for respiratory treatment recommendations. What would you suggest be ordered *at this time*? Why? (The answer should be in the form of *specific* orders.)

———— **PATIENT 2** • **Eddie Shoebridge** ————

PATIENT: Eddie Shoebridge, a fifty-two-year-old male was
            admitted this morning with a diagnosis of
            exacerbation of chronic bronchitis. Patient is alert and
            oriented. He is in a room on a medical-surgical unit.
            He has one peripheral IV.

PHYSICAL
FINDINGS: Pulse 130, BP 146/90, temperature 39°C, respirations
            22, shallow. Breath sounds are decreased in bases with
            rhonchi on exhalation. Frequent productive cough of
            thick, yellow sputum. Patient has a forty pack-year
            smoking history and was smoking a pack a day up to
            admission. Admitting chest x-ray showed bilateral
            basilar infiltrates.

LAB DATA: pH 7.37, $PaCO_2$ 52, PaO_2 54, SaO_2 86%, HCO_3- 29, FiO_2
            0.21. Hgb 18, WBC 14,500.

• • •

The attending physician asks you for respiratory treatment recommendations.
What would you suggest be ordered *at this time*? Why? (The answer should be
in the form of *specific* orders.)

——————— **PATIENT 3** • **Warren Phillips** ———————

PATIENT:

Warren Phillips, a thirty-two-year-old male seen in the emergency department for shortness of breath of rapid onset. Patient has a long history of asthma and is a frequent emergency department visitor. Patient is sitting up in bed in obvious respiratory distress; he has an occasional weak, nonproductive cough. He is wearing a nasal cannula running at 4 Lpm.

PHYSICAL
FINDINGS:

Pulse 110, regular, BP 146/74, temperature 37.4°C, respirations 26, labored. Breath sounds decreased throughout with bilateral expiratory wheezing.

LAB DATA:

SpO_2 94% on nasal cannula at 4 Lpm; no other lab work is done.

• • •

The attending physician asks you for respiratory treatment recommendations. What would you suggest be ordered *at this time*? Why? (The answer should be in the form of *specific* orders.)

--------- **PATIENT 4 • Latisha Jackson** ---------

PATIENT: Latisha Jackson, an eighteen-month-old female seen in the emergency department for acute shortness of breath. Patient is sitting in her mother's lap with obvious shortness of breath. She appears to be well nourished and normal size for her age.

PHYSICAL
FINDINGS: Pulse 126, regular, temperature (rectal) 39°C, respirations 42, labored. Breath sounds decreased with stridor noted on inspiration. Substernal and intercostal retractions noted on inspiration. No coughing or drooling noted. Skin is warm and dry.

LAB DATA: SpO_2 88% on room air. No other lab work was performed.

• • •

The attending physician asks you for respiratory treatment recommendations. What would you suggest be ordered *at this time*? Why? (The answer should be in the form of *specific* orders.)

─────────── **PATIENT 5 • Willie Fremont** ───────────

PATIENT:

Willie Fremont, a sixty-four-year-old male. Patient was admitted six days ago with abdominal pain. He had an aortic aneurysm repair four days ago; was on the ventilator in the surgical intensive care unit for three days post-op. He has recently been transferred to the surgical unit. He is in a regular room with a central line catheter in the jugular vein.

PHYSICAL
FINDINGS:

Pulse 106, regular, BP 146/78, temperature 39.2°C, respirations 24, shallow. Breath sounds decreased with crackles on inspiration in bases. He has an occasional weak, nonproductive cough. Patient has a forty-eight pack-year smoking history; quit smoking six weeks prior to admission. Chest x-ray taken upon discharge from the surgical intensive care unit (SICU) showed some streaky bilateral infiltrates.

LAB DATA:

pH 7.47, $PaCO_2$ 29, PaO_2 54, SaO_2 90%, HCO_3- 21, FiO_2 nasal cannula at 2 Lpm, Hgb 11.3, WBC 13,200.

• • •

The attending physician asks you for respiratory treatment recommendations. What would you suggest be ordered *at this time*? Why? (The answer should be in the form of *specific* orders.)

——————— **PATIENT 6 • Hans Lipper** ———————

PATIENT:

Hans Lipper, a forty-four-year-old male, was admitted this morning with a fever, chills, and substernal pain, histoplasmosis is suspected on the basis of exposure to appropriate conditions. Patient is alert and oriented. He is in a regular room with a peripheral IV.

PHYSICAL
FINDINGS:

Pulse 106, regular, BP 138/60, temperature 38.4°C, respirations 24, slightly labored. Breath sounds decreased, especially in bases with crackles on inspiration, occasional cough, mostly nonproductive. Admitting chest x-ray showed diffuse patchy parenchymal densities.

LAB DATA:

pH 7.48, $PaCO_2$ 32, PaO_2 60, SaO_2 93%, HCO_3- 24, FiO_2 0.21, Hgb 13.8, WBC 12,600.

• • •

The attending physician asks you for respiratory treatment recommendations. What would you suggest be ordered *at this time*? Why? (The answer should be in the form of *specific* orders.)

───── PATIENT 7 • Barry Burnerd ─────

PATIENT:

Barry Burnerd, a forty-two-year-old male. Patient is seen in the intensive care unit. He was on the ventilator for three weeks for flail chest and adult respiratory distress syndrome secondary to chest trauma. Currently, he has a 40% continuous aerosol running through a trach collar over a number 8 Shiley tracheostomy tube. Patient is alert and oriented.

PHYSICAL
FINDINGS:

Pulse 98, regular, BP 140/70, temperature 37.8°C, respirations 24, shallow. Breath sounds decreased throughout with rhonchi on exhalation; occasional weak cough, productive (after suctioning), of small amounts of yellow sputum.

LAB DATA:

pH 7.48, $PaCO_2$ 31, PaO_2 80, SaO_2 96%, HCO_3- 23, FiO_2 0.40, Hgb 12.4, WBC 14,500.

• • •

The attending physician asks you for respiratory treatment recommendations. What would you suggest be ordered *at this time*? Why? (The answer should be in the form of *specific* orders.)

—————— **PATIENT 8 • Pogue McPherson** ——————

PATIENT:

Pogue McPherson, a fifty-six-year-old male admitted for abdominal pain, had a small bowel resection three days ago. Patient is in a regular room on the surgical unit. He is alert and oriented and has a peripheral IV running.

PHYSICAL
FINDINGS:

Pulse 115, regular, BP 162/94, temperature 39.2°C, respirations 26, shallow. Breath sounds are very decreased, especially in the bases; occasional weak, nonproductive cough. Patient is morbidly obese. He has a thirty-four pack-year smoking history; quit six years ago.

LAB DATA:

pH 7.47, $PaCO_2$ 32, PaO_2 51, SaO_2 88% HCO_3- 23, FiO_2 0.21, Hgb 11.4, WBC 12,600.

• • •

The attending physician asks you for respiratory treatment recommendations. What would you suggest be ordered *at this time*? Why? (The answer should be in the form of *specific* orders.)

────────── **PATIENT 9** • **Horace Forest** ──────────

PATIENT: Horace Forest, a forty-year-old male admitted this
                       morning with an acute exacerbation of sarcoidosis.
                       Patient is on a regular unit with a peripheral IV. He is
                       alert and oriented.

PHYSICAL
FINDINGS: Pulse 106, regular, BP 130/80, temperature 38°C,
                       respirations 25, shallow. Breath sounds are decreased
                       in bases with crackles throughout, no coughing.
                       Patient was diagnosed with sarcoidosis six months
                       ago; this is his second hospital admission.

LAB DATA: pH 7.49, $PaCO_2$ 30, PaO_2 56, SaO_2 91%, HCO_3- 22, FiO_2
                       0.21, Hgb 15.3, WBC 11,400.

• • •

The attending physician asks you for respiratory treatment recommendations.
What would you suggest be ordered *at this time*? Why? (The answer should be
in the form of *specific* orders.)

PATIENT 10 • LaWanda Harris

PATIENT: LaWanda Harris, a fifty-six-year-old female was admitted this morning with pneumonia. Patient is on a regular unit and has a peripheral IV running. She is alert and oriented but somewhat sleepy, and wearing a 40% air entrainment mask.

PHYSICAL
FINDINGS: Pulse 88, regular, BP 108/66, temperature 39.2°C, respirations 18, shallow. Breath sounds are very decreased throughout, no coughing. Patient has a forty pack-year smoking history.

LAB DATA: pH 7.27, $PaCO_2$ 75, PaO_2 72, SaO_2 92%, HCO_3- 33, FiO_2 0.40, Hgb 16.4, WBC 12,800.

• • •

The attending physician asks you for respiratory treatment recommendations. What would you suggest be ordered *at this time*? Why? (The answer should be in the form of *specific* orders.)

————— **PATIENT 11** • Mitzi Winston —————

PATIENT:

Mitzi Winston, a twenty-eight-year-old female admitted last night for weakness and what appears to be ascending muscle paralysis. Patient is alert and oriented. She is in a regular room.

PHYSICAL FINDINGS:

Pulse 96, regular, BP 134/82, temperature 37°C, respirations 24, shallow. Breath sounds are decreased throughout, chest expansion is equal but decreased bilaterally. No coughing.

LAB DATA:

pH 7.46, $PaCO_2$ 39, PaO_2 76, SaO_2 96%, HCO_3- 26, FiO_2 0.21, Hgb 14.6, WBC 9,400.

• • •

The attending physician asks you for respiratory treatment recommendations. What would you suggest be ordered *at this time*? Why? (The answer should be in the form of *specific* orders.)

--------- **PATIENT 12 • Homer Folk** ---------

PATIENT:

Homer Folk, a fifty-four-year-old male was admitted last night with congestive heart failure. Patient is in the coronary care unit. He is alert and oriented but a bit anxious. He has a peripheral IV and oxygen via nasal cannula running at 3 Lpm.

PHYSICAL FINDINGS:

Pulse 120, thready, BP 114/60, temperature 36.8°C, respirations shallow, labored. Breath sounds decreased throughout with crackles on inspiration; no coughing. Chest x-ray shows enlarged heart with bilateral vascular congestion. Patient has a history of cardiac exacerbations.

LAB DATA:

pH 7.39, $PaCO_2$ 41, PaO_2 40, SaO_2 75%, HCO_3- 24, FiO_2 via nasal cannula at 3 Lpm, Hgb 15.9, WBC 9,800.

• • •

The attending physician asks you for respiratory treatment recommendations. What would you suggest be ordered *at this time*? Why? (The answer should be in the form of *specific* orders.)

—————— **PATIENT 13** • **B. J. Stooker** ——————

PATIENT: B. J. Stooker, a sixty-year-old male was admitted this
                            morning with a diagnosis of black lung disease.
                            Patient is alert and oriented. He is in a regular room
                            with a peripheral IV.

PHYSICAL
FINDINGS: Pulse 110, regular, BP 136/78, temperature 38.6°C,
                            respirations 28, shallow. Breath sounds are decreased
                            throughout; decreased chest expansion. No coughing.
                            Patient has a forty pack-year smoking history, quit
                            three years ago.

LAB DATA: pH 7.52, $PaCO_2$ 28, PaO_2 54, SaO_2 91%, HCO_3- 22, FiO_2
                            0.21, Hgb 14.8, WBC 6,600.

• • •

The attending physician asks you for respiratory treatment recommendations.
What would you suggest be ordered *at this time*? Why? (The answer should be
in the form of *specific* orders.)

PATIENT 14 • Jack Speck

PATIENT:
Jack Speck, a fifty-four-year-old male was admitted following a closed head injury; had a craniotomy yesterday. Patient is unresponsive, he is in the intensive care unit. He has a central line, a peripheral IV, and an ICP line. He is receiving oxygen by nasal cannula at 6 Lpm.

PHYSICAL
FINDINGS:
Pulse 88, regular, BP 118/68, temperature 38.4°C, respirations 24, shallow. Breath sounds are decreased throughout with crackles in the bases. No coughing. Skin is warm and dry.

LAB DATA:
pH 7.48, $PaCO_2$ 30, PaO_2 64, SaO_2 94%, HCO_3- 22, FiO_2 via nasal cannula at 6 Lpm, Hgb 12.2, WBC 12,300, intercranial pressure (ICP) 18 mm Hg.

• • •

The attending physician asks you for respiratory treatment recommendations. What would you suggest be ordered *at this time*? Why? (The answer should be in the form of *specific* orders.)

—————— **PATIENT 15** • Lucy Minster ——————

PATIENT: Lucy Minster, a ninety-four-year-old female was admitted two days ago from a nursing home for shortness of breath. Patient has a long history of arthritis. She is obtunded and obviously debilitated. She is in a regular room with a peripheral IV.

PHYSICAL
FINDINGS: Pulse 82, thready, BP 94/50, temperature 39°C, respirations 26, shallow. Breath sounds very decreased throughout, weak, nonproductive cough. Skin is warm and dry.

LAB DATA: pH 7.50, $PaCO_2$ 29, PaO_2 47, SaO_2 86%, HCO_3- 23, FiO_2 0.21, Hgb 10.2, WBC 14,300.

• • •

The attending physician asks you for respiratory treatment recommendations. What would you suggest be ordered *at this time*? Why? (The answer should be in the form of *specific* orders.)

——————— **PATIENT 16** • **Ann Felson** ———————

PATIENT:

Ann Felson, a forty-four-year-old female was admitted three days ago for hemoptysis and shortness of breath; had a right thoracotomy yesterday. Patient is in the intensive care unit. She is difficult to arouse. She has a chest tube in the right upper chest draining serosanguinous fluid. She has a nasal cannula running at 6 Lpm.

PHYSICAL
FINDINGS:

Pulse 106, regular, BP 136/84, temperature 38.2°C, respirations 22. Breath sounds decreased over right hemithorax; chest expansion is decreased on the right side. Occasional productive cough of thick red tinged sputum.

LAB DATA:

pH 7.47, $PaCO_2$ 30, PaO_2 74, SaO_2 91%, HCO_3- 22, FiO_2 via nasal cannula 6 Lpm, Hgb 12.4, WBC 11,400.

• • •

The attending physician asks you for respiratory treatment recommendations. What would you suggest be ordered *at this time*? Why? (The answer should be in the form of *specific* orders.)

PATIENT 17 • Leroy Wilson

PATIENT:
Leroy Wilson, a sixty-year-old male was admitted this afternoon for acute shortness of breath of rapid onset. Patient is currently on therapy for squamous-cell lung carcinoma. Patient is alert and anxious. He is in a regular room. He has a peripheral IV and oxygen via nasal cannula at 4 Lpm.

PHYSICAL FINDINGS:
Pulse 120, regular, BP 148/86, temperature 37.4°C, respirations 28, shallow, slightly labored. Breath sounds decreased, especially over the right base; decreased chest expansion over the right base. No coughing. Chest x-ray shows blunted right costophrenic angle.

LAB DATA:
pH 7.51, $PaCO_2$ 28, PaO_2 60, SaO_2 94%, HCO_3^- 22, FiO_2 via nasal cannula at 4 Lpm, Hgb 13.2, WBC 8,800.

• • •

The attending physician asks you for respiratory treatment recommendations. What would you suggest be ordered *at this time*? Why? (The answer should be in the form of *specific* orders.)

—————— **PATIENT 18** • **James Plato** ——————

PATIENT: James Plato, a forty-nine-year-old male was admitted last night with an exacerbation of gastroenteritis and GI bleeding. Patient has a four year history of bronchiectasis. Patient is alert and oriented; he is in the intensive care unit with a nasogastric tube in place.

PHYSICAL
FINDINGS: Pulse 88, regular, BP 114/78, temperature 37.6°C, respirations 22. Breath sounds decreased in bases, with rhonchi on exhalation. Occasional productive cough of thick pale yellow sputum.

LAB DATA: pH 7.38, $PaCO_2$ 52, PaO_2 58, SaO_2 89%, HCO_3- 30, FiO_2 0.21, Hgb 18.2, WBC 9,800.

• • •

The attending physician asks you for respiratory treatment recommendations. What would you suggest be ordered *at this time*? Why? (The answer should be in the form of *specific* orders.)

——————— **PATIENT 19 • Wally Winters** ———————

PATIENT:

Wally Winters, a twenty-two-year-old male was admitted this morning with pneumonia. Patient has a history of cystic fibrosis. He is alert and oriented. He is in a regular room with a peripheral IV and oxygen running at 2 Lpm.

PHYSICAL
FINDINGS:

Pulse 110, regular, BP 110/66, temperature 38.8°C, respirations 24, shallow, slightly labored. Breath sounds decreased throughout with rhonchi on exhalation; chest expansion is decreased in bases. Occasional productive cough of thick, tenacious yellow sputum.

LAB DATA:

pH 7.44, $PaCO_2$ 50, PaO_2 62, SaO_2 93%, HCO_3- 32, FiO_2 via nasal cannula at 2 Lpm, Hgb 16.2, WBC 14,300.

• • •

The attending physician asks you for respiratory treatment recommendations. What would you suggest be ordered *at this time*? Why? (The answer should be in the form of *specific* orders.)

——— PATIENT 20 • Foster Lacey ———

PATIENT: Foster Lacey, a sixty-three-year-old male was admitted this afternoon for a myocardial infarction. Patient has a history of alcohol abuse and liver problems. Patient is alert and oriented; he is in the coronary care unit. He is on a cardiac monitor and has a nasal cannula running at 3 Lpm; he has a peripheral IV.

PHYSICAL
FINDINGS: Pulse 100, some irregular beats, BP 140/92, temperature 37.2°C, respirations 24, slightly labored. Breath sounds are equal bilaterally with fine crackles in bases. No coughing. Skin is warm and moist.

LAB DATA: pH 7.49, $PaCO_2$ 28, PaO_2 56, SaO_2 91%, HCO_3- 20, FiO_2 via nasal cannula at 3 Lpm, Hgb 11.2, WBC 7,800.

• • •

The attending physician asks you for respiratory treatment recommendations. What would you suggest be ordered *at this time*? Why? (The answer should be in the form of *specific* orders.)

————— **PATIENT 21** • **Meredith Fooster** —————

PATIENT: Meredith Fooster, a four-month-old female was
            admitted last night with pneumonia, apparent
            malnutrition, and dehydration. Patient is crying. She is
            on the pediatric unit and has a peripheral IV and a
            nasal cannula running at 2 Lpm.

PHYSICAL
FINDINGS: Pulse 130, regular, temperature (rectal) 41°C,
            respirations 42, labored with intercostal and substernal
            retractions. Breath sounds are decreased with crackles
            on inspiration. She has a frequent loose,
            nonproductive cough. Skin is warm and dry.

LAB DATA: SpO_2 91% on nasal cannula at 2 Lpm.

• • •

The attending physician asks you for respiratory treatment recommendations.
What would you suggest be ordered *at this time*? Why? (The answer should be
in the form of *specific* orders.)

PATIENT 22 • Mandy Mason

PATIENT: Mandy Mason, a nine-month-old female was admitted
                      this morning with a diagnosis of bronchiolitis. Patient
                      is on the pediatric unit. She is alert and crying
                      intermittently. She appears to be well nourished and of
                      normal development for her age.

PHYSICAL
FINDINGS: Pulse 124, regular, temperature 40°C, respirations 40
                      with mild intercostal retractions. Breath sounds are
                      decreased with wheezing on inhalation and
                      exhalation. She has an occasional loose, nonproductive
                      cough. Skin is warm and dry.

LAB DATA: SpO_2 89% on room air.

• • •

The attending physician asks you for respiratory treatment recommendations.
What would you suggest be ordered *at this time*? Why? (The answer should be
in the form of *specific* orders.)

--- **PATIENT 23** • **Sean Wiggins** ---

PATIENT:

Sean Wiggins, a fifty-eight-year-old male was admitted three days ago for acute shortness of breath. Patient had a thoracentesis and bronchoscopy. Cytologic examination revealed a small-cell carcinoma in the lung. Patient is alert and oriented. He is in a regular room with a peripheral IV and oxygen via nasal cannula running at 3 Lpm. Patient has been informed of his diagnosis.

PHYSICAL
FINDINGS:

Pulse 114, regular, BP 138/88, temperature 37.4°C, respirations 24, shallow. Breath sounds are decreased throughout with rhonchi on exhalation in bases. He has an occasional productive cough of thick blood tinged sputum. Patient has a forty-six pack-year smoking history.

LAB DATA:

pH 7.46, $PaCO_2$ 34, PaO_2 62, SaO_2 93%, HCO_3- 22, Hgb 10.7, WBC 11,400.

• • •

The attending physician asks you for respiratory treatment recommendations. What would you suggest be ordered *at this time*? Why? (The answer should be in the form of *specific* orders.)

PATIENT 24 • Willie Lawson

PATIENT:

Willie Lawson, an eighty-five-year-old male. Patient is seen in the home for routine respiratory home care visits. Patient has a long history of COPD and congestive heart failure. He takes the following medication: Lasix, Lanoxin, and Atrovent (2 puffs, q.i.d.). Patient is alert and oriented, and is dressed and out of bed. He has an oxygen concentrator in his home but is not using it at this time.

PHYSICAL
FINDINGS:

Pulse 112, regular, BP 142/90, respirations 26, shallow, slightly labored. Breath sounds are decreased throughout with crackles in bases. He has an occasional weak nonproductive cough. Patient is short of breath at rest and is not able to complete a sentence without stopping to breathe. Skin is warm and moist.

LAB DATA:

SpO_2 86% at rest on room air.

• • •

The attending physician asks you for respiratory treatment recommendations. What would you suggest be ordered *at this time*? Why? (The answer should be in the form of *specific* orders.)

─────── **PATIENT 25** • Neil Armitron ───────

PATIENT: Neil Armitron, a seventy-two-year-old male. Patient is
                            seen in his home for routine home care visits. Patient
                            has a long history of COPD. He takes the following
                            medication: Ativan, Lasix, Atrovent (2 puffs q.i.d.),
                            Proventil (ordered on 2 puffs q.i.d., however, the
                            patient reports typical use of 2 to 4 puffs Q. 2 to 3 h.).
                            Patient is alert, dressed, and out of bed.

PHYSICAL
FINDINGS: Pulse 96, regular, BP 152/88, respirations 24, shallow.
                            Breath sounds are greatly decreased, especially in
                            bases. He has an occasional weak, dry, nonproductive
                            cough. Skin is warm and dry. Patient is thin for his
                            height and reports diminished appetite and a 5 pound
                            weight loss over the past month. He has severe
                            exertional dyspnea; he is not short of breath at rest.

LAB DATA: SpO_2 74% at rest on 4 Lpm via nasal cannula (from a
                            liquid reservoir). Patient has his hematocrit checked
                            every month—last report was 58.

• • •

The attending physician asks you for respiratory treatment recommendations.
What would you suggest be ordered *at this time*? Why? (The answer should be
in the form of *specific* orders.)

CHAPTER FOUR

MECHANICAL VENTILATION

INTRODUCTION

For a variety of reasons, the acuity level of patients in hospitals today is rising. This means that patients need to be monitored more closely. This especially applies to patients with cardiorespiratory pathologies (either primary or secondary).

Although respiratory care practitioners are not ultimately responsible for committing patients to mechanical ventilation, they are often in a position to treat and assess patients with cardiorespiratory compromise. Because of this, the RCP is often asked for recommendations regarding the long term treatment of such patients.

This chapter presents several patient situations in which the patient appears to be developing cardiorespiratory compromise. The learner's task is to analyze each situation and make two of three decisions: 1) should the patient be committed to mechanical ventilation; 2) if so, how should that ventilatory support be implemented (i.e., choice of ventilator, initial settings, etc.); 3) if not, what should be done instead (specific treatment recommendations).

Suggested answers appear at the end of the book. There may be a wide range of opinion about when to actually commit a patient to ventilatory support. The learner must supply specific rationale for decisions. The answers in the book are not meant to be *definitive*, but merely guidelines. In addition, specific ventilator settings are not given. There are various schools of thought as to determining initial ventilator settings. The author tends toward the standard 8 to 10 mL/Kg ideal body weight and a starting FiO_2 of 1.0. It is recognized that other approaches are possible and, in fact, ventilator settings should be specific to the patient and patient condition.

This chapter does not address ventilator management; that will be dealt with in the next chapter.

PATIENT CASES

PATIENT 1 • Arnie Lovelow

PATIENT: Arnie Lovelow, a sixty-two-year old male. He is 69 inches tall, weighs 148 lbs and was admitted two days ago with a diagnosis of emphysema and COPD. Patient is currently difficult to arouse. He is in a regular room, with a peripheral IV running. The difficulty in arousal is a change in his condition. You are seeing him because he is due for aerosol therapy.

PHYSICAL
FINDINGS: Pulse 110, thready, BP 106/52, temperature 37.5°C, respirations 24, slightly labored and shallow. Breath sounds are decreased throughout with rhonchi in lung bases, frequent weak, productive cough of small amounts of thick yellow sputum.

LAB DATA: pH 7.52, $PaCO_2$ 28, PaO_2 48, HCO_3^- 23, SaO_2 87%; patient is on a nasal cannula at 2 Lpm, Hgb 14.2, peak flow 80 Lpm, stat ECG shows sinus tachycardia with occasional PVCs.

CONSIDERATIONS: Patient is currently receiving oxygen via nasal cannula at 2 Lpm. He also gets 0.5cc Proventil in 2.5cc normal saline via aerosol Q. 4h. and Atrovent 2 puffs via MDI q.i.d.

• • •

1. Would you recommend placing this patient on mechanical ventilation?

2. If so, what ventilator and what initial settings would you recommend?

3. If not, what would you recommend be changed or added to his treatment?

———— PATIENT 2 • Mary Gay ————

PATIENT: Mary Gay, a fifty-seven-year-old female is 63 inches tall and weighs 210 lbs. She is being seen in the emergency room for what appears to be an exacerbation of chronic CHF (congestive heart failure). Patient is alert and oriented, but very anxious. You are called to place the patient on a nonrebreathing mask and then draw arterial blood gases (ABGs) in twenty minutes.

PHYSICAL FINDINGS: Pulse 136, thready, BP 110/62, temperature 37°C, respirations 28, shallow and labored. Breath sounds are decreased with coarse crackles on inspiration throughout both lungs. No coughing. Patient is diaphoretic.

LAB DATA: pH 7.34, $PaCO_2$ 46, PaO_2 56, SaO_2 87%, HCO_3- 24, on a nonrebreathing mask; ECG monitor shows sinus tachycardia with widened QRS, occasional abnormal beats.

• • •

1. Would you recommend placing this patient on mechanical ventilation?

2. If so, what ventilator and what initial settings would you recommend?

3. If not, what would you recommend be changed or added to her treatment?

——————— **PATIENT 3 • Filo Bedlam** ———————

PATIENT:

Filo Bedlam, a fifty-year-old male who is 71 inches tall and weighs 200 lbs was admitted this morning with a diagnosis of pneumonia. Patient is difficult to arouse and is a bit confused. He has an IV running and is in a regular room. You are seeing him to administer aerosol therapy.

PHYSICAL
FINDINGS:

Pulse 102, regular, BP 94/40, temperature 40°C, respirations 32, shallow. Breath sounds are decreased in bases with crackles on inspiration, occasional weak, nonproductive cough.

LAB DATA:

pH 7.56, $PaCO_2$ 23, PaO_2 50, SaO_2 88%, HCO_3- 21, FiO_2 40% air entrainment mask, Hgb 12.4, WBC 17,400, chest x-ray (taken this morning) shows bilateral patchy infiltrates in the bases.

CONSIDERATIONS:

Patient is receiving oxygen via 40% air entrainment mask. He has been ordered to receive 0.5cc Proventil in 2.5cc normal saline via small volume nebulizer Q. 3h. followed by postural drainage and percussion.

• • •

1. Would you recommend placing this patient on mechanical ventilation?

2. If so, what ventilator and what initial settings would you recommend?

3. If not, what would you recommend be changed or added to his treatment?

——————— **PATIENT 4** • Jennifer Yaslov ———————

PATIENT:

Jennifer Yaslov, a four-year-old female is 38 inches tall and weighs 42 lbs. Admitted this afternoon with a diagnosis of suspected spinal meningitis. Patient is comatose, responsive only to pain. Patient is in the intensive care unit with two IVs running. You are called to see her to administer oxygen and draw blood gases.

PHYSICAL
FINDINGS:

Pulse 140, regular, BP 82/40, temperature 41°C, respirations 44, shallow, labored (with substernal and intercostal retractions). Breath sounds are decreased throughout. No coughing. Skin is warm and dry with a slight rash covering the extremeties.

LAB DATA:

pH 7.31, $PaCO_2$ 49, PaO_2 50, SaO_2 81%, HCO_3- 23, FiO_2 via nasal cannula at 6 Lpm, Hgb 11.6, WBC 3,400.

• • •

1. Would you recommend placing this patient on mechanical ventilation?

2. If so, what ventilator and what initial settings would you recommend?

3. If not, what would you recommend be changed or added to her treatment?

—————— **PATIENT 5** • **Forrest Grange** ——————

PATIENT:

Forrest Grange, a seventy-year-old male is 70 inches tall, weighs 146 lbs and was admitted four days ago with an exacerbation of bone cancer. Patient is comatose, responsive only to painful stimuli. He is on the oncology ward and is receiving chemotherapy. You are seeing him to draw ABGs.

PHYSICAL
FINDINGS:

Pulse 52, thready, BP 92/40, temperature 37.4°C, respirations 26, shallow. Breath sounds are decreased throughout with crackles in bases. No coughing. Skin is cool and dry.

LAB DATA:

pH 7.24, $PaCO_2$ 60, PaO_2 44, SaO_2 70%, HCO_3- 23, FiO_2 via nonrebreathing mask, Hgb 8.6, WBC 2,400.

CONSIDERATIONS:

Along with the oxygen, the patient receives 0.5cc Proventil in 2.5cc normal saline via aerosol Q. 6h.

• • •

1. Would you recommend placing this patient on mechanical ventilation?

2. If so, what ventilator and what initial settings would you recommend?

3. If not, what would you recommend be changed or added to his treatment?

———— **PATIENT 6** • **Anthony Angle** ————

PATIENT:
Anthony Angle, a ten-year-old male is 52 inches tall and weighs 76 lbs. He was admitted last night with head trauma secondary to a bicycle accident. Patient is in the intensive care unit and is unresponsive. You are seeing him to draw ABGs.

PHYSICAL
FINDINGS:
Pulse 110, regular, BP 96/50, temperature 36.6°C, respirations 38, shallow. Breath sounds are decreased throughout. No coughing.

LAB DATA:
pH 7.22, $PaCO_2$ 58, PaO_2 52, SaO_2 76%, HCO_3- 22, FiO_2 via simple mask at 6 Lpm, Hgb 12.6, ECG monitor shows sinus tachycardia.

CONSIDERATIONS:
Other than oxygen, the patient is receiving no respiratory therapy.

• • •

1. Would you recommend placing this patient on mechanical ventilation?

2. If so, what ventilator and what initial settings would you recommend?

3. If not, what would you recommend be changed or added to his treatment?

—————— **PATIENT 7** • **Pippi Longnecker** ——————

PATIENT: Pippi Longnecker, a seventeen-year-old female is 65
                      inches tall and weighs 126 lbs. Admitted to the
                      intensive care unit from the emergency room for
                      suspected drug overdose (toxicology screen has been
                      requested but not yet completed). Patient is
                      unresponsive. She has a peripheral IV running.

PHYSICAL
FINDINGS: Pulse 52, regular, BP 88/40, temperature 36.4°C,
                      respirations 10, shallow. Breath sounds are decreased
                      throughout. No coughing. Skin is warm and dry.

LAB DATA: pH 7.26, $PaCO_2$ 62, PaO_2 110, SaO_2 96%, HCO_3- 27,
                      FiO_2 via nasal cannula at 4 Lpm, Hgb 14.6. ECG
                      monitor shows sinus rhythm.

CONSIDERATIONS: Other than the oxygen, the patient is receiving no
                      other respiratory therapy at this time.

• • •

1. Would you recommend placing the patient on mechanical ventilation?

2. If so, what ventilator and what initial settings would you recommend?

3. If not, what would you recommend be changed or added to her treatment?

—————— **PATIENT 8** • **John Stryker** ——————

PATIENT:
John Stryker, a sixty-five-year-old male is 73 inches tall and weighs 190 lbs. He was admitted two days ago for liver failure with a history of COPD. Patient is in a monitored bed in the stepdown unit, he is semi-alert. He has a peripheral IV running.

PHYSICAL
FINDINGS:
Pulse 122, thready, BP 148/90, temperature 38.6°C, respirations 26, slightly labored. Breath sounds decreased throughout with rhonchi in the right base, frequent weak, nonproductive cough. Skin is warm and moist.

LAB DATA:
pH 7.32, $PaCO_2$ 56, PaO_2 58, SaO_2 86%, HCO_3- 27, FiO_2 via nasal cannula at 4 Lpm, Hgb 10.2, WBC 3,400. ECG on monitor shows sinus tachycardia with occasional first degree heart block. Chest x-ray (portable, done yesterday) shows basilar infiltrates in both lungs with more on the right.

CONSIDERATIONS:
Along with the oxygen, the patient is receiving 0.5cc Proventil in 2cc 20% mucomyst Q. 4h. with postural drainage and percussion.

• • •

1. Would you recommend placing this patient on mechanical ventilation?

2. If so, what ventilator and what initial settings would you recommend?

3. If not, what would you recommend be changed or added to his treatment?

PATIENT 9 • Sybil Gordon

PATIENT:
Sybil Gordon, a forty-year-old female is 66 inches tall and weighs 156 lbs. She was admitted from the emergency department to the intensive care unit with status asthmaticus. Patient is alert and oriented, but very anxious. She has a peripheral IV running.

PHYSICAL
FINDINGS:
Pulse 136, regular, BP 168/84, temperature 37.2°C, respirations 30, very labored. Breath sounds are very decreased throughout with slight wheezing on exhalation; occasional weak, nonproductive cough. Patient is sitting up, leaning on the bedside table.

LAB DATA:
pH 7.34, $PaCO_2$ 42, PaO_2 48, SaO_2 79%, HCO_3- 22, FiO_2 via nasal cannula at 6 Lpm, Hgb 13.6. Peak flow 60 after three aerosol treatments with 0.5cc Proventil in 2.5cc normal saline.

CONSIDERATIONS:
Along with the oxygen, the patient has received three aerosol treatments in the last hour, she has also received subcutaneous terbutaline and is receiving Solumedrol by IV.

• • •

1. Would you recommend placing this patient on mechanical ventilation?

2. If so, what ventilator and what initial settings would you recommend?

3. If not, what would you recommend be changed or added to her treatment?

——————— **PATIENT 10** • **Baby Girl Gomez** ———————

PATIENT: Baby girl Gomez, a newborn was born an hour ago at
                       thirty weeks gestation (caesarian delivery). Her weight
                       is 1362 grams, Apgar score is 4 at one minute, 5 after
                       five minutes. Patient is in the neonatal intensive care
                       unit. She has a weak cry.

PHYSICAL
FINDINGS: Pulse 130, regular, temperature 36°C, respirations 64
                       with intercostal and substernal retractions. Breath
                       sounds are very decreased with some bronchial
                       sounds over peripheral tissue.

LAB DATA: pH 7.20, $PaCO_2$ 72, PaO_2 40, SaO_2 66%, HCO_3- 26,
                       (umbilical), FiO_2 0.70 (via oxyhood), Hgb 9.6.

CONSIDERATIONS: Other than the oxygen, the patient is receiving no
                       respiratory therapy.

• • •

1. Would you recommend placing this patient on mechanical ventilation?

2. If so, what ventilator and what initial settings would you recommend?

3. If not, what would you recommend be changed or added to her treatment?

―――――― **PATIENT 11** • Anna Clarkstown ――――――

PATIENT:
Anna Clarkstown, an eighty-year-old female is 61 inches tall and weighs 94 lbs. She was admitted two days ago from a nursing home with a diagnosis of pneumonia. Patient is responsive only to painful stimuli. She is in a regular room with a peripheral IV running and a feeding tube in place. You are seeing her to administer routine aerosol therapy.

PHYSICAL
FINDINGS:
Pulse 98, thready, BP 100/48, temperature 39.2°C, respirations 24, shallow. Breath sounds decreased with crackles in bases, occasional weak, nonproductive cough. Skin is warm and dry.

LAB DATA:
pH 7.42, $PaCO_2$ 38, PaO_2 40, SaO_2 76%, HCO_3- 24, FiO_2 via nasal cannula at 4 Lpm, Hgb 10.4, WBC 13,300. Portable chest x-ray from yesterday shows patchy basilar infiltrates in both lungs.

CONSIDERATIONS:
Along with the oxygen, the patient is receiving 0.5cc Proventil in 2.5cc normal saline Q. 4h.

• • •

1. Would you recommend placing this patient on mechanical ventilation?

2. If so, what ventilator and what initial settings would you recommend?

3. If not, what would you recommend be changed or added to her treatment?

PATIENT 12 • Tuco Ramirez

PATIENT:

Tuco Ramirez, a fifty-two-year-old male is 71 inches tall and weighs 210 lbs. He was admitted two hours ago with an exacerbation of myasthenia gravis. Patient is in the intensive care unit with a peripheral IV running. He is alert and oriented. You are seeing him to draw ABGs.

PHYSICAL FINDINGS:

Pulse 102, regular, BP 138/80, temperature 37.1°C, respirations 30, very shallow. Breath sounds are decreased throughout. No coughing. Patient is complaining of some peripheral weakness and dysphagia.

LAB DATA:

pH 7.36, $PaCO_2$ 38, PaO_2 60, SaO_2 90%, HCO_3- 20, FiO_2 0.21, Hgb 13.4, WBC 8,400, positive Tensilon test, peak flow 250 Lpm.

CONSIDERATIONS:

Other than the oxygen, the patient is receiving no respiratory therapy.

• • •

1. Would you recommend placing this patient on mechanical ventilation?

2. If so, what ventilator and what initial settings would you recommend?

3. If not, what would you recommend be changed or added to his treatment?

CHAPTER FIVE

VENTILATOR MANAGEMENT

——— INTRODUCTION ———

In the last chapter, patient situations were presented in which the decision was whether or not to place the patient on mechanical ventilation. The learner was also asked to determine appropriate initial ventilator settings or appropriate alternate therapy.

In this chapter the learner is presented with patients already receiving mechanical ventilation. The learner is given a patient scenario and a ventilator flow sheet. He or she is then asked to determine the best course of action based on the information given. In some cases, some kind of intervention and/or modification might be indicated. In other cases, the best course of action may be to maintain the patient and continue to monitor. In other situations the decision might be made to gather more information before recommending any additional action.

Suggested answers are given at the end of the book.

PATIENT CASES

--------- **PATIENT 1** • **Alvy Singer** ---------

PATIENT: Alvy Singer, a forty-six-year-old male is 68 inches tall,
weighs 132 lbs and was admitted with a diagnosis of
viral pneumonia. The patient was admitted to a
regular room and was receiving fluids and IV
antibiotics when he became unresponsive. ABGs
showed ventilatory failure with severe hypoxemia;
chest x-ray showed complete opacification of the left
side. Approximately fifteen hours after admission, the
decision was made to transfer the patient to the
intensive care unit, intubate, and implement
mechanical ventilation via the P–B 7200. Initial
settings were:
Mode: CMV
Rate: 14 Bpm
V_T: 700 mL
Flow: 60 Lpm
FiO_2:   1.0
Pattern: Square Wave

After intubation and implementation of mechanical ventilation, the patient began
to assist at a rate of 14 breaths per minute (Bpm). Breath sounds indicated rhonchi
over the left side. The patient was suctioned for moderated amounts of thick
yellow sputum. Peak pressure was 42 cm H_2O, plateau pressure was 34 cm H_2O.
Proventil 2 puffs via MDI through the ventilator circuit was ordered. The patient
was placed on the ventilator at 2140 hours on October 12.

It is currently 1700 hours on October 13. The patient is still unresponsive. You are
still suctioning occasional thick yellow sputum. ABGs at 1530 were: pH 7.48,
$PaCO_2$ 29, PaO_2 164, SaO_2 99%, HCO_3- 22.

• • •

Look at the accompanying flow sheet. After examining the information, what
are your recommendations?

SIMULATED MEMORIAL HOSPITAL
VENTILATOR FLOWSHEET

PATIENT DATA Alvy Singer

Age: 46

Type of Ventilator ___P–B 7200___   Date Started ___October 12___

Date	10/12	10/13	10/13		
Time	2140	0800	1700		
Mode	CMV	CMV	CMV		
Set Rate	14 Bpm	14 Bpm	14 Bpm		
Pt Rate	14 Bpm	14 Bpm	16 Bpm		
V_T Set	700mL	700mL	700mL		
V_T Returned	690mL	685mL	692mL		
Spont V_T	—	—	—		
Total V_E	9.8L	9.8L	11.2L		
Flow	60 Lpm	60 Lpm	60 Lpm		
Waveform	Square	Square	Square		
FiO_2	1.0	.80	.60		
PEEP/CPAP	—	—	—		
Insp Time (%)	—	—	—		
Press Supp	—	—	—		
Peak Press	42 cm H_2O	39 cm H_2O	41 cm H_2O		
Plat Press	34 cm H_2O	30 cm H_2O	30 cm H_2O		
Press Limit	60 cm H_2O	60 cm H_2O	60 cm H_2O		
Humidity	HME	HME	HME		
Other					

Patient Monitoring Parameters

Heart Rate	110	112	114		
BP	110/60	116/62	118/64		
S_PO_2	100%	100%	99%		
Breath Sound	bilateral/rhonchi	bilateral/rhonchi	bilateral/rhonchi		
ABGs		7.48/32/192	7.48/29/164		
Other					

Comments: number 8 endotracheal (ET) tube

———— **PATIENT 2** • **Samantha Eastway** ————

PATIENT: Samantha Eastway, a twenty-six-year-old female is 63 inches tall, weighs 164 lbs and was admitted through the emergency department with an acute asthma episode. In the emergency department she received six aerosol treatments with albuterol, subcutaneous terbutaline, IV Solu-medrol, and oxygen via nasal cannula at 6 Lpm. After four hours her peak flow was less than 100. She began to get confused and poorly responsive, and her breath sounds became greatly diminished throughout. Her arterial blood gases showed increasing $PaCO_2$ and moderate hypoxemia. The decision was made to admit her to the intensive care unit (ICU), intubate her, and place her on mechanical ventilation. In the ICU she was given Valium and vancuronium. She was intubated and placed on the P–B 7200 with the following settings:

Mode: CMV
Rate: 16 Bpm
V_T: 600 mL
Flow: 50 Lpm
FiO_2:   60%
Pattern: decelerating

After the patient was established on the ventilator, her breath sounds were increased with a prolonged expiratory phase. Her peak pressure was 48 cm H_2O; plateau pressure was 26 cm H_2O. Proventil 2 puffs via MDI through the ventilator circuit was ordered Q. 1h. x 6. The patient was placed on the ventilator at 1935 hours on November 1.

It is currently 1350 hours on November 2. The patient is still being heavily sedated. Breath sounds are still somewhat diminished with some expiratory wheezing noted. ABGs at 1230 were pH 7.36, $PaCO_2$ 44, PaO_2 78, SaO_2 95%, HCO_3- 25.

• • •

Look at the accompanying flow sheet. After examining the information, what are your recommendations?

SIMULATED MEMORIAL HOSPITAL VENTILATOR FLOWSHEET

PATIENT DATA Samantha Eastway
Age: 26

Type of Ventilator ___P–B 7200___   Date Started ___November 1___

Date	11/1	11/1	11/2		
Time	1940	2300	1230		
Mode	CMV	CMV	CMV		
Set Rate	16 Bpm	16 Bpm	16 Bpm		
Pt Rate	—	—	—		
V_T Set	600mL	600mL	600mL		
V_T Returned	580mL	572mL	566mL		
Spont V_T	—	—	—		
Total V_E	9.6L	9.6L	9.6L		
Flow	50 Lpm	50 Lpm	50 Lpm		
Waveform	decelerating	decelerating	decelerating		
FiO_2	60%	50%	50%		
PEEP/CPAP	—	—	—		
Insp Time (%)	—	—	—		
Press Supp	—	—	—		
Peak Press	48 cm H_2O	52 cm H_2O	54 cm H_2O		
Plat Press	26 cm H_2O	27 cm H_2O	29 cm H_2O		
Press Limit	65 cm H_2O	65 cm H_2O	65 cm H_2O		
Humidity	HME	HME	HME		
Other					

Patient Monitoring Parameters

Heart Rate	120	102	106		
BP	146/90	130/84	128/86		
SpO_2	97%	96%	95%		
Breath Sound	very diminished	very diminished	slight expiratory wheeze		
ABGs	—	—	7.36/44/78		
Other	—	—	—		

Comments: number 7.5 ET tube   patient is paralyzed

——————— **PATIENT 3** • **Bertha Ferrentino** ———————

PATIENT:

Bertha Ferrentino, a seventy-year-old female is 61 inches tall, weighs 110 lbs and was admitted with an acute exacerbation of COPD. She has a sixty pack-year smoking history, and was still smoking up to admission. The patient was admitted to a regular room, and IV antibiotics were started along with Aminophylline IV, Atrovent 2 puffs via MDI q.i.d., and aerosol therapy with albuterol Q. 4h. She was placed on oxygen via nasal cannula at 2 Lpm. Chest x-ray showed bilateral basilar infiltrates and some widening of the costophrenic angles; the heart was slightly enlarged. Arterial blood gases showed the patient to be a CO_2 retainer. About twelve hours after admission, she began to show signs of clinical deterioration. Her respirations became more labored and shallow, and she became less responsive; her ABGs showed ventilatory failure. At this point, the decision was made to transfer her to the intensive care unit, intubate, and place her on mechanical ventilation. Initial settings on the Servo 900C were:

Mode: SIMV
V_E: 8.4 L
Rate: 10 Bpm
FiO_2:   50%
Pattern: Square Wave

After intubation and implementation of mechanical ventilation the patient had a spontaneous respiratory rate of 16 and a spontaneous V_T of 150 mL (average). Breath sounds were decreased, especially in the bases, with a prolonged expiratory phase. Peak pressure was 38 cm H_2O; plateau pressure was 22 cm H_2O. Albuterol via small volume nebulizer was ordered through the ventilator circuit Q. 4h. The patient was placed on the ventilator at 2245 hours on April 15.

It is currently 1300 hours on April 18. The patient is alert and oriented. Breath sounds are still decreased in the bases. ABGs drawn at 0730 were: pH 7.44, $PaCO_2$ 46, PaO_2 68, SaO_2 94%, HCO_3- 31.

• • •

Look at the accompanying flow sheet. After examining the information, what are your recommendations?

SIMULATED MEMORIAL HOSPITAL VENTILATOR FLOWSHEET

PATIENT DATA   Bertha Ferrentino

Age: 70

Type of Ventilator ___Servo 900C___   Date Started ___April 15___

Date	4/15	4/16	4/18		
Time	2245	1800	1300		
Mode	SIMV	SIMV	SIMV		
Set Rate	10 Bpm	8 Bpm	6 Bpm		
Pt Rate	16 Bpm	14 Bpm	16 Bpm		
V_T Set	840mL	840mL	840mL		
V_T Returned	810mL	815mL	808mL		
Spont V_T	150ml	220ml	240ml		
Total V_E	10.8 Lpm	9.8 Lpm	9.5 Lpm		
Flow	—	—	—		
Waveform	Square	Square	Square		
FiO_2	50%	40%	35%		
PEEP/CPAP	—	—	—		
Insp Time (%)	25%	25%	25%		
Press Supp	—	—	—		
Peak Press	38 cm H_2O	42 cm H_2O	36 cm H_2O		
Plat Press	22 cm H_2O	26 cm H_2O	24 cm H_2O		
Press Limit	60 cm H_2O	60 cm H_2O	60 cm H_2O		
Humidity	HME	HME	HME		
Other	—	—	—		

Patient Monitoring Parameters

Heart Rate	110	96	88		
BP	148/90	132/88	126/84		
S_PO_2	98%	98%	95%		
Breath Sound	diminished with rhonchi	diminished with rhonchi	diminished with rhonchi		
ABGs	—	—	7.44/46/68		
Other					

Comments:

PATIENT 4 • Anton Garcia

PATIENT:

Anton Garcia, a thirty-six-year-old male is 73 inches tall, weighs 210 lbs and was admitted with a diagnosis of pancreatitis and pneumonia. The patient was initially admitted to the intensive care unit (ICU) for close observation. Approximately four hours after admission, the patient became less responsive; respirations became rapid and shallow; ECG showed sinus tachycardia. ABGs showed a low PaO_2 on a nonrebreather mask and an increasing $PaCO_2$; SpO_2 was 86%. The chest x-ray showed increasing bilateral opacification with some vascular engorgement eminating from the hilum. At this point it was thought that the patient was developing adult respiratory distress syndrome and the decision was made to intubate him and place him on mechanical ventilation. Initial settings on the P–B 7200a were:

Mode: CMV
Rate: 16 Bpm
V_T: 900 mL
Flow: 50 Lpm
FiO_2:   1.0
PEEP: +5 cm H_2O
Pattern: Square Wave

The patient was sedated. Breath sounds were equal bilaterally, with some bronchial sounds heard over peripheral lung tissue. Peak pressure was 54 cm H_2O, plateau pressure was 47 cm H_2O. The patient was placed on the ventilator at 1930 hours on January 23.

It is currently 1040 hours on January 25. The patient is still being sedated. Breath sounds are equal bilaterally. Occasionally, he is suctioned for moderate amounts of frothy white sputum. ABGs at 0700 were pH 7.33, $PaCO_2$ 49, PaO_2 82, SaO_2 95%, HCO_3- 26. The patient has a Swan-Ganz catheter in place: readings from an hour ago show a cardiac output of 3.8 L and a pulmonary capillary wedge pressure (PCWP) of 28 mm Hg.

• • •

Look at the accompanying flow sheet. After examining the information, what are your recommendations?

SIMULATED MEMORIAL HOSPITAL
VENTILATOR FLOWSHEET

PATIENT DATA Anton Garcia

Age: 36

Type of Ventilator ___P–B 7200a___   Date Started ___January 23___

Date	1/23	1/24	1/25		
Time	1930	1100	1040		
Mode	CMV	CMV	CMV		
Set Rate	16 Bpm	16 Bpm	16 Bpm		
Pt Rate	0	0	0		
V_T Set	900mL	900mL	900mL		
V_T Returned	898mL	902mL	901mL		
Spont V_T	—	—	—		
Total V_E	14.4 Lpm	14.4 Lpm	14.4 Lpm		
Flow	50 Lpm	45 Lpm	45 Lpm		
Waveform	Square	Square	Square		
FiO_2	1.0	.90	.90		
PEEP/CPAP	+5 cm H_2O	+10 cm H_2O	+10 cm H_2O		
Insp Time (%)	—	—	—		
Press Supp	—	—	—		
Peak Press	54 cm H_2O	58 cm H_2O	62 cm H_2O		
Plat Press	47 cm H_2O	51 cm H_2O	53 cm H_2O		
Press Limit	65 cm H_2O	70 cm H_2O	75 cm H_2O		
Humidity	HME	HME	HME		
Other	—	—	—		

Patient Monitoring Parameters

Heart Rate	112	108	114		
BP	108/60	106/58	104/56		
S_PO_2	95%	94%	92%		
Breath Sound	some broncheal	clear diminished	clear diminished		
ABGs	—	—	—		
Other					

Comments:

───────── **PATIENT 5** • Samuel Peppercorn ─────────

PATIENT:

Samuel Peppercorn, a twenty-two-year-old male is 74 inches tall, weighs 235 lbs and was admitted through the emergency department (via surgery) to the surgical intensive care unit following a stab wound to the chest. The wound is in the right upper chest and was made with scissors. The patient has a chest tube in the right upper chest draining serosanguinous fluid. He is sedated and on ventilatory support. Breath sounds are slightly decreased on the right side with no adventitious sounds. Ventilator settings on the Servo 900C are:

Mode:	Volume Control
Rate:	12 Bpm
V_E:	10.6 Lpm
Inspired time:	25%
FiO_2:	1.0
Pattern:	Square Wave

The patient was not assisting due to heavy sedation. Peak pressure was 46 cm H_2O, plateau pressure was 37 cm H_2O. Initial mechanical ventilation was established at 0230 hours on March 2.

It is currently 2150 hours on March 2. The patient is emerging from sedation and is showing some agitation with increased work of breathing. Chest x-ray showed good aeration on the left side with some infiltrates on the right side. ABGs done at 2000 were pH 7.48, $PaCO_2$ 26, PaO_2 264, SaO_2 99%, HCO_3- 19.

• • •

Look at the accompanying flow sheet. After examining the information, what are your recommendations?

SIMULATED MEMORIAL HOSPITAL VENTILATOR FLOWSHEET

PATIENT DATA Samuel Peppercorn
Age: 22

Type of Ventilator __Servo 900C__   Date Started __March 2__

Date	3/2	3/2	3/2		
Time	0230	0900	2200		
Mode	VC	VC	VC		
Set Rate	12 Bpm	12 Bpm	12 Bpm		
Pt Rate	—	—	—		
V_T Set	880mL	880mL	880mL		
V_T Returned	870mL	865mL	875mL		
Spont V_T	—	—	—		
Total V_E	10.6 Lpm	10.6 Lpm	10.6 Lpm		
Flow	—				
Waveform	Square	Square	Square		
FiO_2	1.0	1.0	1.0		
PEEP/CPAP	—	—	—		
Insp Time (%)	25%	25%	25%		
Press Supp	—	—	—		
Peak Press	46 cm H_2O	43 cm H_2O	39 cm H_2O		
Plat Press	37 cm H_2O	35 cm H_2O	30 cm H_2O		
Press Limit	65 cm H_2O	65 cm H_2O	65 cm H_2O		
Humidity	Cascade	Cascade	Cascade		
Other	—	—	—		

Patient Monitoring Parameters

Heart Rate	94	90	92		
BP	98/60	104/62	108/62		
S_PO_2	95%	94%	92%		
Breath Sound	decreased on right	decreased on right	decreased on right		
ABGs	—	—	7.48/26/264		
Other					

Comments:

─────────── **PATIENT 6 • Freda Watkins** ───────────

PATIENT:

Freda Watkins, a fifty-year-old female is 64 inches tall, weighs 190 lbs and was admitted with severe chest pain. Patient had emergency coronary artery bypass surgery twelve hours after admission. She has a thirty pack-year smoking history and has been diagnosed with COPD. She came out of surgery to the surgical intensive care unit on a P–B 7200 ventilator. She was not assisting at all. Breath sounds were equal bilaterally with some crackles noted in the bases. Ventilator settings were:

Mode: CMV
Rate: 14 Bpm
V_T: 700 mL
Flow: 50 Lpm
FiO_2:   1.0
Pattern: Square Wave

Peak pressure was 38 cm H_2O, plateau pressure was 24 cm H_2O. The patient was placed on the ventilator at 1950 hours on April 18.

It is now 1620 hours on April 20; the patient is alert and oriented, although still being given Demerol for pain. Breath sounds are equal bilaterally with some rhonchi on exhalation. She is assisting the ventilator. ABGs done at 1200 hours were pH 7.46, $PaCO_2$ 34, PaO_2 118, SaO_2 98%, HCO_3- 24. AM chest x-ray showed some slight vascular engorgement and a slight flattening of the costophrenic angles. Cardiac output is 4.2 L.

• • •

Look at the accompanying flow sheet. After examining the information, what are your recommendations?

SIMULATED MEMORIAL HOSPITAL VENTILATOR FLOWSHEET

PATIENT DATA   Freda Watkins
Age: 50

Type of Ventilator _____P–B 7200_____   Date Started _April 18_

Date	4/18	4/19	4/20		
Time	2000	1400	1620		
Mode	CMV	CMV	CMV		
Set Rate	14 Bpm	12 Bpm	12 Bpm		
Pt Rate	—	14 Bpm	16 Bpm		
V_T Set	700mL	700mL	700mL		
V_T Returned	700mL	700mL	700mL		
Spont V_T	—	—	—		
Total V_E	9.8 Lpm	9.8 Lpm	11.2 Lpm		
Flow	50 Lpm	50 Lpm	50 Lpm		
Waveform	Square	Square	Square		
FiO_2	1.0	0.70	0.60		
PEEP/CPAP	—	—	—		
Insp Time (%)	—	—	—		
Press Supp	—	—	—		
Peak Press	38 cm H_2O	36 cm H_2O	34 cm H_2O		
Plat Press	24 cm H_2O	28 cm H_2O	26 cm H_2O		
Press Limit	60 cm H_2O	60 cm H_2O	60 cm H_2O		
Humidity	HME	HME	HME		
Other	—	—	—		

Patient Monitoring Parameters

Heart Rate	110	102	98		
BP	114/70	118/72	124/80		
S_PO_2	99%	99%	98%		
Breath Sound	crackles in bases	clear	rhonchi in bases		
ABGs					
Other					

Comments:

PATIENT 7 • Lorita Menendez

PATIENT:

Lorita Menendez, a thirty-five-year-old female is 66 inches tall, weighs 126 lbs and was admitted with a diagnosis of possible Guillain-Barré Syndrome. Because of increasing muscle weakness, decreasing peak flows, and increasing $PaCO_2$ levels, the patient was intubated and placed on ventilator support. All prior medical history was negative. Initial ventilator settings on the P–B 7200 were:

Mode: CMV
Rate: 12 Bpm
V_T: 700 mL
Flow: 60 Lpm
FiO_2:   40%
Pattern: decelerating

After the ventilator was established the patient was sedated. Her breath sounds were equal bilaterally with no adventitious sounds. Her peak pressure was 26 cm H_2O, plateau pressure was 20 cm H_2O. Ventilation was established at 1820 hours on May 1.

It is now 0900 hours on May 20. The patient is showing some signs of extremity movement and does attempt to assist on occasion. Breath sounds are equal bilaterally with some rhonchi on exhalation. Chest x-ray is clear. ABGs done at 0700 show pH 7.44, $PaCO_2$ 39, PaO_2 98, SaO_2 97%, HCO_3- 25.

• • •

Look at the accompanying flow sheet. After examining the information, what recommendations do you have?

SIMULATED MEMORIAL HOSPITAL VENTILATOR FLOWSHEET

PATIENT DATA Lorita Menendez

Age: 35

Type of Ventilator ___P–B 7200___   Date Started ___May 1___

Date	5/1	5/20			
Time	1820	0900			
Mode	CMV	CMV			
Set Rate	12 Bpm	12 Bpm			
Pt Rate	—	13 Bpm			
V_T Set	700mL	700mL			
V_T Returned	700mL	700mL			
Spont V_T	—	—			
Total V_E	8.4 Lpm	9.1 Lpm			
Flow	60 Lpm	60 Lpm			
Waveform	decelerating	decelerating			
FiO_2	40%	30%			
PEEP/CPAP	—	—			
Insp Time (%)	—	—			
Press Supp	—	—			
Peak Press	26 cm H_2O	30 cm H_2O			
Plat Press	20 cm H_2O	22 cm H_2O			
Press Limit	50 cm H_2O	50 cm H_2O			
Humidity	HME	HME			
Other					

Patient Monitoring Parameters

Heart Rate	96	102			
BP	122/80	130/82			
S_PO_2	99%	97%			
Breath Sound	clear	rhonchi			
ABGs		7.44/39/98			
Other					

Comments: number 8.0 ET Tube

——————— **PATIENT 8** • **Joseph Abramowitz** ———————

PATIENT:

Joseph Abramowitz, a sixty-two-year-old male is 69 inches tall, weighs 184 lbs and was admitted to the hospital for abdominal surgery. He has a long history of COPD. Patient developed serious wound infection twenty-four hours post-operatively. He then became septic and went into septic shock and ventilatory failure. He was placed on the ventilator. Even though the wound healed after three weeks, and the sepsis cleared, the patient could not be weaned from the ventilator. Once he became medically stable, he was transferred to a subacute care facility.

Upon admission to the subacute care facility, he was placed on a Aequitron LP–6 ventilator with the following settings:

Mode:	Assist/Control
Rate:	10 Bpm
V_T:	700 mL
Inspiratory time:	1.2 sec
FiO_2:	5 L bleed-in

The patient was alert and oriented on admission. Breath sounds were clear and diminished in the bases. Peak pressure was 36 cm H_2O. The patient was suctioned occasionally for moderate amounts of thick white sputum. He was assisting at a rate of 14 Bpm to 16 Bpm. Proventil and Atrovent, 2 puffs Q. 6h. through the ventilator was initiated. Admission to the subacute care facility was at 1300 hours on August 20.

It is now 0900 hours on August 23. The patient is now assisting at a rate of 16 Bpm to 18 Bpm. Peak pressure is between 38 cm H_2O and 44 cm H_2O. The patient is complaining of being short of breath occasionally. The breath sounds are still equal bilaterally, very decreased in the bases. A small amount of thick yellow sputum is being suctioned from the tracheostomy tube.

• • •

Look at the accompanying flow sheet. After examining the information, what are your recommendations?

SIMULATED MEMORIAL HOSPITAL VENTILATOR FLOWSHEET

PATIENT DATA Joseph Abramowitz

Age: 62

Type of Ventilator ___LP–6___   Date Started ___August 20___

Date	8/20	8/23			
Time	1300	0900			
Mode	A/C	A/C			
Set Rate	10 Bpm	10 Bpm			
Pt Rate	14 Bpm	16 Bpm			
V_T Set	700mL	700mL			
V_T Returned	—	—			
Spont V_T	—	—			
Total V_E	9.6 Lpm	11.2 Lpm			
Flow	—	—			
Waveform					
FiO_2	5 L bleed-in	5 L bleed-in			
PEEP/CPAP	—	—			
Insp Time (%)	1.2 seconds	1.2 seconds			
Press Supp	—	—			
Peak Press	36 cm H_2O	40 cm H_2O			
Plat Press	—	—			
Press Limit	60 cm H_2O	60 cm H_2O			
Humidity	HME	HME			
Other					

Patient Monitoring Parameters

Heart Rate	86	102			
BP	134/90	144/92			
S_PO_2	98%	95%			
Breath Sound	clear	very decreased			
ABGs					
Other					

Comments:

──────── **PATIENT 9** • Nellie Wanamaker ────────

PATIENT: Nellie Wanamaker, a eighty-four-year-old female is 62
            inches tall, weighs 110 lbs and was originally admitted
            to the hospital from a nursing home with a diagnosis
            of pneumonia and osteoarthritis. Two days after
            admission, the patient developed ventilatory failure
            and was given ventilatory support. After a week the
            pneumonia seemed to clear, but the patient could not
            be weaned from the ventilator. After two weeks the
            patient became stable enough to transfer to the
            subacute care facility. She was admitted to the
            subacute care facility at 1500 hours on September 20.
            She was placed on the Aequitron LP-6 on the
            following settings:
            Mode: IMV
            Rate: 8 Bpm
            V_T: 600mL
            Inspiratory time: 1.0 sec
            FiO_2:   4 L bleed-in

Upon admission, the patient was unresponsive to all but painful stimuli; her
spontaneous respiratory rate was 10 Bpm; her spontaneous V_T was 150 mL to 250
mL. Peak pressures were 36 cm H_2O. Breath sounds were decreased throughout
with some crackles heard in the bases. She was suctioned occasionally for small
amounts of thick pale yellow sputum.

It is now 0900 hours on September 28; the patient's physical and clinical status has
not changed since admission.

• • •

Look at the accompanying flow sheet. What recommendations do you have?

SIMULATED MEMORIAL HOSPITAL VENTILATOR FLOWSHEET

PATIENT DATA Nellie Wanamaker

Age: 84

Type of Ventilator __LP–6__   Date Started __September 20__

Date	9/20	9/28			
Time	1500	0900			
Mode	IMV	IMV			
Set Rate	8 Bpm	8 Bpm			
Pt Rate	10 Bpm	12 Bpm			
V_T Set	600mL	600mL			
V_T Returned	—	—			
Spont V_T	200 mL	150=250 mL			
Total V_E	6.8 Lpm	6.6 Lpm			
Flow	—	—			
Waveform	—	—			
FiO_2	4 L bleed-in	4 L bleed-in			
PEEP/CPAP	—	—			
Insp Time (%)	1.0 seconds	1.0 seconds			
Press Supp	—	—			
Peak Press	36 cm H_2O	38 cm H_2O			
Plat Press	—	—			
Press Limit	55 cm H_2O	55 cm H_2O			
Humidity	HME	HME			
Other					

Patient Monitoring Parameters

Heart Rate	92	98			
BP	112/70	110/68			
S_PO_2	96%	93%			
Breath Sound	decreased with crackles in bases	decreased with crackles in bases			
ABGs					
Other					

Comments:

——————— **PATIENT 10** • Nolan Sanchez ———————

PATIENT: Nolan Sanchez, a one-month-old male; weight is 4 Kg. The patient was brought to the emergency room by his father who noted that he was pale with labored breathing and a decreased activity level. Until admission the child was in apparent good health except for a car accident approximately thirty hours ago. Upon admission it was noted that the patient was a well developed one month old with moderate respiratory distress. Respiratory rate was 50 with moderate intercostal and substernal retractions. Breath sounds were clear, heart rate 180, blood pressure 72/49, temperature 36°C. Bruises to the orbits, right scalp, and back were noted. The neurological exam was normal. Chest x-ray showed fractures to the left humerus, three ribs, and the left femur; there was also a basilar skull fracture. SpO_2 was 96% on 50% oxygen. The patient was admitted for multiple trauma. An hour after admission, the patient was intubated with a number 3.5 endotracheal tube and placed on mechanical ventilation in order to control intracranial pressure. Dilantin was given to control seizures. Settings on the Servo 900C were:

Mode: SIMV
Rate: 15 Bpm
V_T: 10.8 cc/Kg
I:E ratio: 1:4.3
PEEP: +4 cm H_2O
FiO_2:   .30

Mechanical ventilation was established on 2130 hours October 15.

It is now 1300 hours on October 16. The patient is paralyzed to slow seizure activity. Breath sounds are equal and clear bilaterally. Chest rise is good. Arterial blood gases at 1000 are pH 7.29, $PaCO_2$ 41, PaO_2 103, SaO_2 97%, HCO_3- 19.

• • •

Look at the accompanying flow sheet. After examining the information, what are your recommendations?

SIMULATED MEMORIAL HOSPITAL
VENTILATOR FLOWSHEET

PATIENT DATA   Nolan Sanchez

Age: 1 month

Type of Ventilator ___Servo 900C___   Date Started __October 15__

Date	10/15	10/15	10/16		
Time	2130	2310	1300		
Mode	SIMV	SIMV	SIMV		
Set Rate	15 Bpm	18 Bpm	16 Bpm		
Pt Rate	10 Bpm	18 Bpm	16 Bpm		
V_T Set	10.81 cc/kg	42	38		
V_T Returned	41 mL	42 mL	37 mL		
Spont V_T	—	—	—		
Total V_E	—	—	—		
Flow	—	—	—		
Waveform	Square	Square	Square		
FiO_2	0.30	0.40	0.30		
PEEP/CPAP	+4 cm H_2O	+4 cm H_2O	+4 cm H_2O		
Insp Time (%)	25%	20%	25%		
Press Supp	—	—	—		
Peak Press	18 cm H_2O	19 cm H_2O	19 cm H_2O		
Plat Press	13 cm H_2O	14 cm H_2O	15 cm H_2O		
Press Limit	25 cm H_2O	25 cm H_2O	25 cm H_2O		
Humidity	HME	HME	HME		
Other					

Patient Monitoring Parameters

Heart Rate	182	170	149		
BP	—	—	70/34		
S_PO_2	100%	100%	100%		
Breath Sound	clear	clear	clear		
ABGs	—	7.42/26/212	7.29/41/103		
Other					

Comments: 10/15, 2300—patient is paralyzed, respirations increased to 18

——————— **PATIENT 11** • **Baby Boy Francini** ———————

PATIENT:

Baby Boy Francini, a full term, 4.8 Kg neonate, born ten minutes ago to a thirty-four-year-old gravida 6, para 1 mother with pregnancy induced diabetes. The patient was delivered by caesarian section. At delivery tenacious meconium was suctioned from below the vocal cords. Apgars were 5, 7, and 7. Pulse was 141, temperature 36.1°C, respiratory rate about 90 Bpm, with increasing respiratory distress manifested by grunting, nasal flaring, and intercostal and substernal retractions. Chest x-ray showed bilateral fluffy infiltrates. Breath sounds were equal bilaterally with scattered crackles on inspiration. Due to increasing $PaCO_2$ and decreasing PaO_2 on 50% oxygen, the patient was intubated and placed on ventilatory support. Settings on the Bear Cub were:

Mode:	IMV
Rate:	40 Bpm
Flow:	10 Lpm
PIP:	25cm H_2O
I:E:	1:2
FiO_2:	1.0
PEEP:	+5cm H_2O

After being placed on the ventilator, the patient ceased all ventilatory effort. Chest rise was equal bilaterally; breath sounds were diminished. Mechanical ventilation was established at 0430 hours on June 14.

It is now 1530 on June 14. One hour after a dose of Survanta, the patient has good chest rise; breath sounds are equal bilaterally with scattered crackles. Color is pink. Arterial blood gases done thirty minutes after the study are pH 7.32, $PaCO_2$ 45, PaO_2 139, SaO_2 99%, HCO_3- 22.

• • •

Look at the accompanying flow sheet. After examining the information, what recommendations do you have?

SIMULATED MEMORIAL HOSPITAL VENTILATOR FLOWSHEET

PATIENT DATA Baby Boy Francini

Age: Newborn

Type of Ventilator _Bear Cub_   Date Started _June 14_

Date	6/14	6/14	6/15		
Time	0430	1530	0200		
Mode	IMV	IMV	IMV		
Set Rate	40 Bpm	50 Bpm	50 Bpm		
Pt Rate	0	0	0		
V_T Set	—	—	—		
V_T Returned	—	—	—		
Spont V_T					
Total V_E	—	—	—		
Flow	10 Lpm	10 Lpm	10 Lpm		
Waveform	—	—	—		
FiO_2	1.0	1.0	1.0		
PEEP/CPAP	+5 cm H_2O	+5 cm H_2O	+5 cm H_2O		
Insp Time (%)	0.8	0.7	0.7		
Press Supp	—	—	—		
Peak Press	—	—	—		
Plat Press	—	—	—		
Press Limit	25 cm H_2O	30 cm H_2O	30 cm H_2O		
Humidity	Concha	Concha	Concha		
Other			p̄ Survanta		

Patient Monitoring Parameters

Heart Rate	145	140	150		
BP	—	—	—		
S_PO_2	100%	100%	100%		
Breath Sound	diminished	diminished	crackles		
ABGs	7.35/46/65	7.35/47/81	7.32/45/139		
Other	good chest rise	—	good chest rise		

Comments: number 3 ET tube

─────── **PATIENT 12 • Baby Girl Hank** ───────

PATIENT:

Baby Girl Hank, a twenty-six week (gestation), 870 gram neonate, born to a twenty-six-year-old gravida 8, para 4 mother with no prenatal care and a history of substance abuse. The patient was born via caesarian section due to breech presentation. Immediately after birth, she was limp and blue. She was intubated immediately. The heart rate was below 100 beats per minute. CPR was started and epinepherine was given via endotracheal tube. After two minutes, heart rate was over 100 and the CPR was stopped. After five minutes, the pulse was 140 beats per minute, temperature 35°C, respiratory rate (spontaneous) zero. Breath sounds equal bilaterally with scattered crackles. The patient was placed on the Bear Cub with the following settings:

Mode: IMV
Rate: 40 Bpm
PIP: 28cm H_2O
Flow: 8 Lpm
I:E ratio: 1:1.4
FiO_2:   1.0
PEEP: +6 cm H_2O

After ventilatory support was established, the chest rise was good and equal bilaterally. The patient was placed on the ventilator at 0510 hours on July 20.

It is now 1440 hours on July 20. Chest rise is still good bilaterally; breath sounds are equal with some crackles, especially in the bases. Arterial (umbilical) blood gases are pH 7.24, $PaCO_2$ 52, PaO_2 59, SaO_2 90%, HCO_3- 21.

• • •

Look at the accompanying flow sheet. After examining the data, what recommendations do you have?

SIMULATED MEMORIAL HOSPITAL VENTILATOR FLOWSHEET

PATIENT DATA Baby Girl Hank

Age: Newborn

Type of Ventilator ___Bear Cub___   Date Started _July 20_

Date	7/20	7/20			
Time	0510	1400			
Mode	IMV	IMV			
Set Rate	40 Bpm	40 Bpm			
Pt Rate	0	20 Bmp			
V_T Set	—	—			
V_T Returned	—	—			
Spont V_T	—	—			
Total V_E	—	—			
Flow	8 Lpm	9 Lpm			
Waveform	—	—			
FiO_2	1.0	.90			
PEEP/CPAP	+6 cm H_2O	+6 cm H_2O			
Insp Time (%)	.6	.6			
Press Supp	—	—			
Peak Press	—	—			
Plat Press	—	—			
Press Limit	28 cm H_2O	26 cm H_2O			
Humidity	Concha	Concha			
Other					

Patient Monitoring Parameters

Heart Rate	140	149			
BP	—	—			
S_PO_2	95%	91%			
Breath Sound	crackles	crackles			
ABGs	7.37/44/53	7.24/52/59			
Other	good chest rise	chest rise good			

Comments:

CHAPTER SIX

CLINICAL SITUATIONS

— INTRODUCTION —

During the course of a work period, a respiratory care practitioner might encounter a variety of situations that are out of the ordinary or are unanticipated. This chapter will present the learner with a number of such situations that will require immediate action. As is the custom, *loose* answers will be provided at the end of the book; however, because these are isolated situations, many possible approaches may exist. Specific answers should attempt to consider all possible contingencies and should contain rationale.

Clinical Situation 1

You are the only therapist assigned to the night shift of a 150-bed suburban hospital. It is 0200 hours; you are making treatment rounds when you hear the code signal announcing a cardiac arrest in the intensive care unit (ICU). You rush to the scene and begin establishing ventilation via bag and mask. Five minutes into the code, it becomes apparent that the patient will need to be intubated. As you prepare to intubate, another code is announced for the emergency department.

How do you handle this situation?

Clinical Situation 2

You are assigned to do oxygen rounds on the second shift in a 200-bed suburban hospital. You remove the flowmeter from the wall outlet of a patient whose oxygen has been discontinued. As you remove the flowmeter from the wall outlet, you are surprised by a massive leak of oxygen from the wall outlet, as though the outlet did not close after the flowmeter was removed. Oxygen is filling the room and the noise is deafening.

How do you handle this situation?

Clinical Situation 3

You are assigned to take call and perform all ABGs and ECGs on the day shift of a 150-bed rural hospital. You receive a call from the emergency department to do a stat ECG on a patient with a chest pain. On the way to the emergency department you receive another stat call for ABGs on a patient in respiratory distress on one of the nursing units.

How do you handle this situation?

Clinical Situation 4

You are assigned to perform floor therapy on the evening shift of a 250-bed urban hospital. You are administering aerosol therapy to your patient; suddenly you realize that the patient in the other bed is anxious and appears to be in moderate respiratory distress. This patient is not on the respiratory service and you do not know anything about him.

What do you do?

Clinical Situation 5

You are assigned to perform floor therapy on the night shift in a 500-bed teaching hospital. You enter the patient's room to perform aerosol therapy. The patient has been unresponsive in the past. As you proceed to administer the aerosol, you observe that the patient is not breathing. She has a weak pulse, about 30 beats per minute; her skin is warm to the touch. She has a diagnosis of bone cancer that has metastisized to the brain. Her code status is unknown.

What do you do?

Clinical Situation 6

You are assigned to perform floor therapy on the day shift of a 300-bed urban hospital. You receive an order to begin incentive spirometry on a patient who had a thoracotomy yesterday. Upon reviewing the patient's chart you find that the preliminary tissue report suggests predominantly small-cell carcinoma. Chest x-ray shows small masses throughout both lungs. You enter the patient's room and begin explaining the procedure. The patient asks if he has cancer and if he is terminal.

How do you answer the patient?

Clinical Situation 7

You are assigned to the sixteen bed step-down unit in a 600-bed university hospital. You are checking the ventilator of a patient with amyotrophic lateral sclerosis. The patient has been on the ventilator for six weeks. The attending physician summons you away from the bedside. She explains that the patient and the family have expressed a desire to end the ventilatory support via terminal wean. The physician indicates that she is going to begin a morphine drip. She wants you to gradually decrease the rate on the ventilator, and remove the ventilator once the patient is asleep.

How do you handle this situation?

Clinical Situation 8

You are making your second home visit to a patient who is receiving oxygen via nasal cannula at 2 Lpm. The oxygen is coming from a concentrator in the next room. The patient has a long history of COPD, and his SpO_2 on room air is 86%. As you enter the house, you find that the patient is smoking with the oxygen in place.

What do you do about the situation?

Clinical Situation 9

It is 2130 hours on a Saturday night. An electrical storm has disrupted power for part of the city. You receive a call from a home patient indicating that his concentrator is not working and his back up E cylinder has only 500 psi remaining. He is normally on a nasal cannula running at 3 Lpm. He wants to know what to do in case the power is not soon restored.

What do you tell him?

Clinical Situation 10

You are making a visit to a patient who is receiving oxygen via nasal cannula at 2 Lpm. The patient has a liquid reservoir in the home and has a transfillable-portable. She indicates that she wants to visit relatives who live 250 miles away. She will be traveling by car to their location. She wants to know what she can do about her oxygen.

What do you tell her?

Clinical Situation 11

You are consulting at a 100-bed skilled nursing facility. You are informed that a patient is being admitted with a tracheostomy tube in place. She is to receive oxygen via the tracheostomy at 35%. The facility does not have wall oxygen or compressed air, and primarily uses concentrators for oxygen delivery.

How do you set this up?

Clinical Situation 12

You are working the night shift at a fifty-bed skilled nursing facility with a five-bed ventilator unit. The nurse calls you to see a patient, stating that the patient is complaining of shortness of breath. The patient is alert and oriented, and is receiving ventilatory support via a Aequitron LP–6 ventilator with a 3 Lpm oxygen bleed in. The patient appears to be in respiratory distress with increased work of breathing.

What do you do?

CHAPTER SEVEN

EXTENDED CLINICAL SITUATIONS

──── INTRODUCTION ────

The second (and perhaps most challenging) portion of the Registry Examination process is the clinical simulation exam. One of the problems in preparing for this exam is that there are few sample simulations written at a level understandable to students not close to graduation. This chapter presents several simple extended clinical situations in a format similar to the Clinical Simulation Exam administered by the NBRC.

The purpose of this chapter is to expose the learner to the process of gathering information and making appropriate therapeutic decisions based on that information. Obviously, this book does not match the actual test conditions (e.g., latent image technology, various pathways to completion, etc.); several good sources are already available that match the actual exam (see References). The answers only indicate appropriateness, they are not scored. For final preparation for the actual clinical simulation, the learner is referred to the NBRC self-assessment exams and/or the several test-preparation workshops offered around the country.

EXTENDED SITUATION 1
Amanda Rottwiler

Part A

You are working the day shift in a 300-bed suburban hospital. You get a call from the floor indicating that Amanda Rottwiler is going for a CT scan. She will require oxygen both for the transport and during the scan. You are asked to assist with the transport. What items of information will you need to insure a successful transport? (*You may select as many as you feel are indicated*)

1. vital signs

2. diagnosis

3. age

4. arterial blood gases

5. SpO_2

6. current oxygen therapy

7. breath sounds

8. general appearance

9. pulmonary function results

10. chest x-ray

11. procedure to be performed in CT scan

Part B

Based on the information given, how do you handle the situation? (*Select only one*)

1. Place on nasal cannula at 4 Lpm; transport on E cylinder

2. Keep on 35% air entrainment mask at 6 Lpm; transport on E cylinder

3. Place on nasal cannula at 6 Lpm; transport on M cylinder

4. Place on nasal cannula at 10 Lpm; transport on M cylinder

Part C

The procedure and transport should take about 75 minutes. You are transporting on an E cylinder with 1800 lbs pressure. How many minutes remain if 4 Lpm of oxygen is used?

1. 94 minutes

2. 126 minutes

3. 158 minutes

4. 204 minutes

EXTENDED SITUATION 2
Mohammad Omann

Part A

You are working the evening shift of a 226-bed community hospital. You receive a stat page to the emergency department to see a patient described by the nurse as being in severe respiratory distress. As you enter the patient's cubicle, you observe a middle-age adult male in severe respiratory distress. The patient is leaning forward on a bedside table, breathing rapidly with marked use of accessory muscles. Breath sounds are very decreased with very faint wheezing superimposed over a prolonged expiratory phase. Your first response to this patient would be to: (*Select only one*)

1. Place the patient on a 0.30 air entrainment mask with ABGs after thirty minutes

2. Place the patient on a nonrebreather mask and do a complete assessment

3. Administer stat IPPB with 0.5cc Albuterol in 2.5cc normal saline

4. Administer stat aerosol treatment with 0.5cc Isoetharine in 2.5cc normal saline

5. Administer stat aerosol treatment with 20mg Intal in 2.0cc normal saline

Part B

An hour later, the patient has had three consecutive aerosol treatments as well as subcutaneous epinephrine. He is still short of breath and the doctor wants you to evaluate the patient further and recommend further action. You would evaluate the following: (*You may select as many as you feel necessary*)

1. medications taken at home

2. gag reflex

3. arterial blood gases

4. breath sounds

5. appearance of chest

6. heart sounds

7. methacholine challenge

8. ECG

9. vital signs

10. sputum culture & sensitivity

11. history of lung disease

12. CBC

13. chest x-ray

14. lung scan

15. P_50

16. pulmonary function test

17. peak flow

18. history of present illness

Part C

It is now ninety minutes later and the patient has had two more aerosol treatments. The doctor informs you that the patient is going to be admitted and asks for your recommendations for an appropriate treatment regimen. You would recommend: (*You may select as many as you feel appropriate*)

1. IV theophylline

2. aerosol treatments with 0.5cc albuterol in 2.5cc normal saline Q. 6h. while awake

3.   arterial blood gases Q. 2h.

4. O_2 by nasal cannula at 2 Lpm

5. aerosol treatments with 0.5cc albuterol in 2.5cc normal saline Q. 2h. x 4 then Q. 4h.

6. IPPB with 0.5cc Bronkosol in 2.5cc normal saline Q. 4h.

7. chest physiotherapy after each aerosol treatment

8. peak flow before and after each aerosol treatment

9. oxygen via 0.50 air entrainment mask

10. incentive spirometry Q. 1h. while awake

Part D

Thirty minutes later, arterial blood gases on 0.50 air entrainment mask reveal:

$$pH\ 7.48,\ PaCO_2\ 27,\ PaO_2\ 58,\ HCO_3\text{-}\ 19,\ SaO_2\ 88\%$$

The physician requests that you place the patient on a nonrebreather mask and repeat ABGs in one hour. You would: (*Select only one*)

1. Place patient on nonrebreather mask and draw ABGs in one hour.

2. Suggest to the physician that too much oxygen can be harmful to the patient and recommend maintaining the current oxygen therapy.

3. Recommend intubation and mechanical ventilation.

4. Give the patient a stat aerosol treatment with albuterol.

Part E

One hour later, arterial blood gases on the nonrebreather mask reveal:

$$pH\ 7.47,\ PaCO_2\ 30,\ PaO_2\ 189,\ HCO_3\text{-}\ 20,\ SaO_2\ 99\%$$

You would now recommend: (*Select only one*)

1. maintaining current oxygen therapy

2. intubation and mechanical ventilation

3. decreasing the oxygen to nasal cannula at 6 Lpm

4. noninvasive pressure support ventilation

Part F

It is now two days later. The patient is doing well; lungs are clear and respiratory distress is minimal. Arterial blood gases on nasal cannula at 2 Lpm show:

$$pH\ 7.41,\ PaCO_2\ 38,\ PaO_2\ 110,\ HCO_3\text{-}\ 23,\ SaO_2\ 98\%$$

The physician asks for your recommendations for home therapy. You would recommend: (*You may select as many as you feel are appropriate*)

1. chest physiotherapy q.i.d.

2. 2 puffs Intal q.i.d.

3. 2 puffs albuterol q.i.d.

4. 40 mg prednisone Q.d

5. 2 puffs flunisolide b.i.d.

6. oxygen via nasal cannula 2 Lpm

7. asthma education

EXTENDED SITUATION 3
Kalyanna Shimatsu

Part A

You are assigned to the ten-bed intensive care unit of a 300-bed teaching hospital. Suddenly the nurse assigned to Kalyanna Shimatsu signals you. She asks you to increase the FiO_2 on the Puritan–Bennett 7200 from 50% to 100% because the patient's heart rate is dropping. Your first reaction would be to: (*Select only one*)

1. Make the change as ordered.
2. Have the nurse contact the attending physician for an order.
3. Call your supervisor.
4. Perform a quick assessment of the situation.

Part B

In order to perform an assessment appropriate for the situation, you would gather which of the following pieces of information? (*Select as many as you feel are necessary*)

1. general appearance
2. breath sounds
3. temperature
4. arterial blood gases
5. heart rate
6. chest x-ray
7. ventilator settings
8. peak airway pressure
9. exhaled tidal volume
10. diagnosis
11. ECG
12. SpO_2

Part C

Once you have assessed the patient, the most appropriate course of action would be to: (*Select only one*)

1. Make the oxygen change as requested.
2. Call the physician to see the patient.
3. Remove the patient from the ventilator and manually ventilate.
4. Increase the tidal volume on the ventilator.

Part D

The patient is now off the ventilator. The nurse is manually ventilating and reports that the patient is 'difficult to bag.' The patient continues to lose consciousness. The SpO_2 has increased from 74% to 80%. The most appropriate course of action would be to: (*Select only one*)

1. Gather information about the ventilator function (perform an EST).
2. Lavage and suction the patient.
3. Insert a number 14 angiocath in the anterior chest.
4. Call for a new ventilator.

Part E

The lavage and suctioning produces a large amount of very thick yellow sputum. The heart rate is increasing, the SpO_2 is now 92% five minutes after the procedure. The nurse reports that is now easier to bag the patient. The most appropriate course of action would be to: (*Select only one*)

1. Continue to bag and suction.
2. Place the patient back on the ventilator on the original settings.
3. Call the patient's physician for further instructions.
4. Change the FiO_2 on the ventilator to 100%.

EXTENDED SITUATION 4
Sanford Williams

Part A

You are the RCP assigned to the emergency department on the evening shift of a 400-bed urban hospital. You are called to see Sanford Williams, an elderly male rescued from a house fire. You arrive just as the patient is being brought in by the paramedics. He is minimally alert and apparently confused. His face is covered with smoke residue. His breathing pattern is rapid and shallow. The physician asks you to initiate the most appropriate therapy at this time. You would: (*Select only one*)

1. Place him on a nonrebreather mask.
2. Place him on a nasal cannula at 6 Lpm.
3. Place him on a simple mask at 8 Lpm.
4. Administer 0.5mL albuterol in 3mL normal saline via small volume nebulizer.

Part B

Once therapy is initiated, you are asked to recommend what items of information would help to determine a future therapeutic course. (*Select as many as you feel are appropriate*)

1. arterial blood gases
2. pulse oximetry
3. co-oximetry
4. gag reflex
5. auscultation
6. vital signs
7. ECG
8. lateral neck x-rays
9. lung scan
10. portable chest x-ray
11. sputum culture & sensitivity
12. medical history
13. general appearance

Part C

During the course of the exam the patient has become less responsive; respiratory rate is still rapid and shallow. You would now recommend: (*Select only one*)

1. intubation and mechanical ventilation
2. intubation and CPAP at 5 cm H_2O and 100% O_2
3. additional aerosol therapy with albuterol
4. maintain present therapy

—— EXTENDED SITUATION 5 ——
Jamal Phelps

Part A

You are the resident respiratory therapist at a camp for asthmatic children. It is mid-afternoon and you get a call from a counselor that Jamal Phelps, a ten-year-old male, became short of breath during a game of "Capture the Flag." He is now resting quietly in the shade but is still complaining of shortness of breath. He does not have an inhaler with him. You decide to see him in the field. You should take the following with you: (*Select as many as you feel are appropriate*)

1. oxygen tank and mask
2. Ventolin inhaler
3. Intal inhaler
4. Azmacort inhaler
5. pulse oximeter
6. portable aerosol machine and albuterol solution (unit dose)
7. stethoscope
8. sphygmomanometer
9. injectable epinepherine
10. peak flowmeter

Part B

You arrive at the scene and find Jamal sitting under a tree. You would now assess the following: (*Select as many as you feel are appropriate*)

1. breath sounds
2. general appearance
3. skin color
4. capillary refill
5. pupillary reaction
6. SpO_2
7. blood pressure
8. heart rate
9. respiratory rate
10. peak flow

Part C

On the basis of your assessment, you would do which of the following: (*Select only one*)

1. Administer 2 puffs of Ventolin via metered dose inhaler and observe.
2. Administer 2 puffs Azmacort via metered dose inhaler and observe.
3. Transport him back to the camp clinic for treatment.
4. Call for EMS backup.
5. Offer no immediate treatment but observe him for 15 minutes.

Part D

Six hours later, Jamal is complaining of increased shortness of breath upon returning to the lodge area following a campfire. You would assess: (*Select as many as you feel are appropriate*)

1. general appearance
2. breath sounds
3. blood pressure
4. SpO_2
5. peak flow
6. heart rate
7. respiratory rate
8. skin color
9. capillary refill time
10. temperature

Part E

Based on your assessment, you would do which of the following: (*Select as many as you feel are appropriate*)

1. Administer 200mg of Theo–Dur.
2. Administer 40mg of oral prednisone.
3. Inject 0.3mg of epinepherine.
4. Administer 0.5mL Ventolin in 2.5mL normal saline via small volume nebulizer every twenty minutes times three.
5. Administer 2 puffs of Intal.
6. Call for EMS backup.
7. Administer oxygen via mask at 5 Lpm.

EXTENDED SITUATION 6
Maya Inunu

Part A

You are working the evening shift at a 400 bed urban medical center. You receive a call to obtain arterial blood gases on Maya Inunu, a patient who has just been admitted from the emergency department. What equipment should you bring with you to obtain the arterial blood? (*Select as many as you feel are appropriate*)

1. heparinized syringe
2. 10cc waste syringe
3. one 23 gauge, 1 inch needle
4. one 20 gauge 1 1/2 inch needle
5. Betadine swabs
6. sterile gauze
7. bandages
8. needle cutter
9. gloves
10. gown
11. mask
12. alcohol prep pads

Part B

What information do you need about the patient? (*Select as many as you feel are appropriate*)

1. name
2. temperature
3. diagnosis
4. prothrombin time and partial thromboplastin time
5. medical history
6. oxygen use and device
7. medications presently used
8. most recent arterial blood gas results

9. electrolytes

10. hemoglobin

Part C

You draw the arterial blood without incident. Once analyzed, you obtain the following results:

pH	7.37	
$PaCO_2$	56 mm Hg	
HCO_3-	31 mEq	
PaO_2	68 mm Hg	
SaO_2	93%	

You should do which of the following once you have obtained the results? (*Select only one*)

1. Call the patient's physician immediately.
2. Phone the results to the unit secretary.
3. Fax the results to the unit.
4. Report the results to the patient's nurse.

Part D

Fifteen minutes later you get an order to change the oxygen to a 40% air entrainment mask. You would do which of the following: (*Select only one*)

1. Increase the oxygen via nasal cannula to 4 Lpm.
2. Recommend changing to a nonrebreathing mask.
3. Implement the order as stated.
4. Perform your own assessment of the patient.

Part E

You would assess which of the following: (*Select as many as you feel are appropriate*)

1. general appearance
2. SpO_2
3. breath sounds
4. peak flow
5. mental status
6. nature of cough

7. heart rate

8. respiratory rate

9. amount of chest expansion

10. chest x-ray

Part F

On the basis of your assessment, you would recommend which of the following? (*Select only one*)

1. Administer oxygen via a 50% air entrainment mask.

2. Implement order as previously written.

3. Leave oxygen as it is (maintain nasal cannula at 3 Lpm).

4. Recommend changing to a 28% air entrainment mask.

5. Recommend instituting mechanical ventilation.

EXTENDED SITUATION 7
Maime Mast

Part A

You are the on-call therapist for a small, suburban, home medical equipment dealer. You receive a call from the visiting nurse for Maime Mast, a seventy-nine-year old female. The nurse indicates that Ms Mast has been having trouble breathing and the nurse wants you to assess the patient and make recommendations for additional therapy, if necessary. Ms Mast's principal diagnosis is COPD, and she has an oxygen concentrator in her home. Upon arrival at her home, you would assess which of the following? (*Select as many as you feel are appropriate*)

1. blood pressure

2. temperature

3. mental status

4. general appearance

5. peak flow

6. breath sounds

7. presence of peripheral edema

8. heart rate

9. sputum production

10. SpO_2

11. chest expansion

12. respiratory rate

13. activity level

14. medications currently being taken and compliance

Part B

On the basis of your assessment, you would recommend which of the following: (*Select as many as you feel are appropriate*)

1. nocturnal oxygen study

2. complete arterial blood gases

3. nasotracheal suction

4. increase oxygen to 4 Lpm

5. Pulmoaide nebulizer with unit dose albuterol q.i.d. and p.r.n.

6. oral suction with a Yankauer

7. flunisolide (Aerobid) via MDI, 2 puffs, b.i.d.

8. admission to the hospital

Part C

The appropriate equipment has been delivered to the home. Ms Mast's daughter, Jan, will be the primary caregiver. Which of the following should Jan be taught? (*Select as many as you feel are appropriate*)

1. appropriate cleaning procedures for suction and nebulizer equipment

2. chest auscultation

3. monitoring sputum for color changes

4. medication side effects

5. suctioning technique

6. blood pressure measurement

Part D

Two weeks later you get a call from Jan indicating that Ms Mast seems to be more dyspneic and less alert than before. Based on this conversation and the wishes of Ms Mast and her family, it is decided not to call EMS, but rather have you visit the patient as soon as possible (the physician has authorized you to make p.r.n. visits). Upon arrival you would assess which of the following: (*Select as many as you feel are appropriate*)

1. SpO_2

2. temperature

3. general appearance

4. recent activity

5. concentrator function

6. Pulmoaide function

7. suction machine function

8. blood pressure

9. breath sounds

10. nature of sputum

Part E

On the basis of your assessment, you would do which of the following? (*Select only one*)

1. Obtain a new concentrator.
2. Recommend increasing the frequency of the aerosol treatments to Q. 3h.
3. Recommend adding chest clapping.
4. Recommend hospital admission.
5. Recommend further assessment.

CHAPTER EIGHT

EXERCISES

━━━━━ INTRODUCTION ━━━━━

As opposed to the other chapters in which the learner used data along with other patient related information to guide clinical decision making, this chapter deals strictly with the manipulation of data—calculations and interpretations. The material will be patient related but the learner will only manipulate the numbers, not make any clinical decisions. The exercises will involve the areas of blood gases, pulmonary function, hemodynamics, and pharmacology. As always, solutions are provided at the end of the book.

SECTION ONE • Blood Gas Analysis

In this section, the learner will be confronted with a number of patient scenarios. Each of these scenarios will contain blood gas data along with other items of information. The learner will be required to interpret the data, both in terms of labeling the arterial blood gas portion of the data and in stating how each data point deviates from accepted normals. The learner will then be required to make a number of calculations based on the data.

Scenario One

The patient is a sixty-one-year-old male admitted with convulsions. CT scan revealed no hematoma or active hemorrhage. After admission the patient developed bilateral pneumonia. The chest x-ray just prior to intubation revealed diffuse patchy infiltrates bilaterally, more severe in the right base.

Data

pH	7.41	PO_2	107 mm Hg	Na^+	142 mEq
$PaCO_2$	38 mm Hg	SaO_2	96%	K^+	2.6 mEq
HCO_3-	24 mEq	Hb	6.9 gm%	Cl^-	97 mEq
PvO_2	48 mm Hg	SvO_2	82%	Glucose	22
(Puritan–Bennett 7200:		A/C, rate 12, V_T 600mL, FiO_2 0.80)			
P_B	740 mm Hg	P_ECO_2	32 mm Hg		

Questions

1. Interpret the arterial blood gas (including the oxygenation state).

2. Interpret the other values.

3. Calculate the following:

   a. anion gap

   b. $P(A\text{-}a)O_2$

   c. CaO_2

   d. $C(a\text{-}v)O_2$

   e. V_D/V_T

   f. Q_S/Q_T

Scenario Two

The patient is a seventy-year-old female, admitted with acute shortness of breath and a history of COPD and pneumonia.

Data

pH	7.637	PaO_2	109 mm Hg	Na^+	143 mEq
$PaCO_2$	21 mm Hg	SaO_2	95%	K^+	3.9 mEq
$HCO_3\text{-}$	23 mEq	Hgb	9.2 gm%	Cl^-	110 mEq
FiO_2	0.40 air entrainment mask			P_B	750 mm Hg

Questions

1. Interpret the arterial blood gas (including the oxygentation state).

2. Interpret the other values.

3. Calculate the following:

   a. anion gap

   b. $P(A-a)O_2$

   c. CaO_2

Scenario Three

The patient is a sixty-eight-year-old female, very obese; admitted and placed on the ventilator for acute ventilatory failure.

Data

pH	7.48	PaO_2	82 mm Hg	Na^+	138 mEq
$PaCO_2$	46 mm Hg	SaO_2	94%	K+	4.3 mEq
HCO_3-	34 mEq	Hgb	7.9 gm%	Cl^-	95 mEq
PvO_2	36 mm Hg	SvO_2	73%	P_B	745 mm Hg
$PECO_2$	36 mm Hg				

(Puritan-Bennett 7200: A/C, rate 10, V_T 700 mL, FiO_2 0.50)

Questions

1. Interpret the arterial blood gas (including the oxygenation state).

2. Interpret the other values.

3. Calculate the following:

  a. anion gap

  b. $P(A\text{-}a)O_2$

  c. CaO_2

  d. $C(a\text{-}v)O_2$

  e. V_D/V_T

  f. Q_S/Q_T

Scenario Four

The patient is a seventy-eight-year-old female admitted with chief complaints of dyspnea and vaginal bleeding. Chest x-ray showed bilateral pleural effusion. The patient has a productive cough of a moderate amount of straw colored sputum. She is diagnosed with malignant tumors in her lungs and abdomen.

Data

pH	7.43	PaO_2	78 mm Hg	Na^+	142 mEq
$PaCO_2$	48 mm Hg	SaO_2	90%	K^+	4.0 mEq
HCO_3^-	31 mEq	Hgb	11.7 gm%	Cl^-	101 mEq
FiO_2	0.35 air entrainment mask			P_B	735 mm Hg

Questions

1. Interpret the arterial blood gases (including the oxygenation state).

2. Interpret the other values.

3. Calculate the following:

   a. anion gap

   b. $P(A-a)O_2$

   c. CaO_2

Scenario Five

The patient is a forty-two-year-old male admitted to the emergency department via squad car after being found unconscious. The patient is a known diabetic. He has bilateral rhonchi.

Data

pH	7.33	PaO_2	224 mm Hg	Na^+	148 mEq
$PaCO_2$	35 mm Hg	SaO_2	96%	K^+	4.1 mEq
HCO_3-	18 mEq	Hgb	9.5 gm%	Cl^-	119 mEq
FiO_2	0.50 aerosol mask			P_B	750 mm Hg

Questions

1. Interpret the arterial blood gas (including the oxygenation state).

2. Interpret the other values.

3. Calculate the following:

   a. anion gap

   b. $P(A-a)O_2$

   c. CaO_2

Scenario Six

The patient is a sixty-four-year-old female admitted with severe respiratory distress and weak productive cough of small amounts of thick, yellow sputum. After admission, arterial blood gases showed acute ventilatory failure; she was placed on the ventilator.

Data

pH	7.437	PaO_2	141 mm Hg	Na^+	139 mEq
$PaCO_2$	33 mm Hg	SaO_2	97%	K^+	3.2 mEq
HCO_3-	23 mEq	Hgb	13.7 gm%	Cl^-	109 mEq
PvO_2	32 mm Hg	SvO_2	64%	P_B	734 mm Hg
P_ECO_2	20 mm Hg				

[Puritan–Bennett 7200: A/C, rate 14, V_T 500 mL, FiO_2 0.50]

Questions

1. Interpret the arterial blood gas (including the oxygenation state).

2. Interpret the other values.

3. Calculate the following:

   a. anion gap

   b. $P(A\text{-}a)O_2$

   c. CaO_2

   d. $C(a\text{-}v)O_2$

   e. V_D/V_T

   f. Q_S/Q_T

SECTION TWO • Hemodynamics

In this section, the learner will be confronted with patient scenarios which contain a hemodynamic profile. The learner will then be required to interpret the data in terms of how the values deviate from normal. In addition, the learner will make a number of calculations based on the data.

Scenario One

The patient is a fifty-six-year-old male who was originally admitted following a head injury. The patient subsequently had a craniotomy and was returned to the surgical intensive care unit on a ventilator. Currently, he is receiving nitroprusside and dobutamine. His chest x-ray is essentially clear.

Data

pH	7.46	PaO_2	121 mm Hg	SaO_2	99%
$PaCO_2$	32 mm Hg	HCO_3-	23 mEq	Hgb	12.4 gm%
Heart Rate	88 beats/min	SBP	156/51	PAP	36/20
PCWP	10	CVP	5 mm Hg	CO	4.9 Lpm

(SIMV: rate 10, V_T 600mL, FiO_2 0.50, P_{peak} 25 cm H_2O, $P_{plateau}$ 16 cm H_2O)

Patient: 70 inches tall, 180 lbs

Questions

1. Interpret the data.

2. Calculate the following:

   a. stroke volume

   b. cardiac index

c. left ventricular stroke work

d. right ventricular stroke work

e. systemic vascular resistance

f. pulmonary vascular resistance

g. static compliance

h. airway resistance

Scenario Two

The patient is a sixty-year-old male admitted with cancer of the esophagus. The patient subsequently had an esophagogastrectomy. He has a history of COPD, coronary artery disease, hypertension, and mycardial infarction. Following surgery he was placed on the ventilator and was receiving Lasix, KCl, Impenem, Flagyl, Digoxin, Verapamil, $MgSO_4$, Vanomycin, and Tobramycin. The chest x-ray shows bilateral pulmonary edema with some consolidation in the left base. The sputum shows Serratia marcescens.

Data

pH	7.47	PaO_2	500 mm Hg	SaO_2	100%
$PaCO_2$	29 mm Hg	HCO_3-	18 mEq	Hgb	10.4 gm%
Heart Rate	95 beats/min	SBP	159/79	PAP	34/12
PCWP	12	CVP	7 mm Hg	CO	4.7 Lpm

(SIMV: rate 12, V_T 800 mL, FiO_2 1.0, P_{peak} 28 cm H_2O, $P_{plateau}$ 19 cm H_2O)

Patient: 69 inches tall, 210 lbs

Questions

1. Interpret the data.

2. Calculate the following:

   a. stroke volume

   b. cardiac index

   c. left ventricular stroke work

   d. right ventricular stroke work

   e. system vascular resistance

   f. pulmonary vascular resistance

   g. static compliance

   h. airway resistance

   i. oxygen delivery

   j. oxygen consumption

Scenario Three

The patient is a fifty-four-year-old female admitted with ischemic heart disease. The patient underwent angioplasty and sustained a dissection of one of her coronary arteries during the procedure. This required emergency coronary artery bypass surgery. After surgery, the patient remained on mechanical ventilation and required an intra-aortic balloon pump. Her medications include epinepherine, dobutamine, and Ancef.

Data

pH	7.34	PaO_2	64 mm Hg	SaO_2	87%
$PaCO_2$	43 mm Hg	HCO_3-	23 mEq	Hgb	8.4 gm%
Heart Rate	127 beats/min	SBP	88/53	PAP	50/32
PCWP	15	CVP	20 mm Hg	Q_T	4.0 Lpm

(SIMV: rate 10, V_T 1000 mL, FiO_2 0.70, PEEP +5 cm H_2O, P_{peak} 30 cm H_2O, $P_{plateau}$ 24)

Patient: 64 inches tall, 146 lbs

Questions

1. Interpret the data.

2. Calculate the following:

   a. stroke volume

   b. cardiac index

   c. left ventricular stroke work

   d. right ventricular stroke work

   e. systemic vascular resistance

   f. pulmonary vascular resistance

   g. static compliance

   h. airway resistance

   i. oxygen delivery

   j. oxygen consumption

Scenario Four

The patient is a seventy-two-year-old female admitted for acute ventilatory failure and congestive heart failure. The patient also has a urinary tract infection and a history of pulmonary hypertension and mitral valve stenosis. Her medications include: Digoxin, KCl, Thiamine, and Lasix. Her chest x-ray shows interstitial pulmonary infiltration and cardiomegaly.

Data

pH	7.49	PaO_2	170 mm Hg	SaO_2	99%
$PaCO_2$	33 mm Hg	HCO_3-	25 mEq	Hgb	14.8 gm%
Heart rate	70 beats/min	SBP	101/48	PAP	67/25
PCWP	18	CVP	17 mm Hg	Q_T	5.7 Lpm

(SIMV: rate 8, V_T 800 mL, FiO_2 0.35, +10 pressure support, P_{peak} 55 cm H_2O, $P_{plateau}$ 45)

Patient: 61 inches tall, 110 lbs

Questions

1. Interpret the data.

2. Calculate the following:

   a. stroke volume

   b. cardiac index

   c. left ventricular stroke work

   d. right ventricular stroke work

   e. systemic vascular resistance

   f. pulmonary vascular resistance

   g. static compliance

   h. airway resistance

   i. oxygen delivery

   j. oxygen consumption

SECTION THREE • Pulmonary Function Interpretation

In this section, the learner will be confronted with patient scenarios accompanied by pulmonary function data, including relevant graphs. The learner will then be required to interpret the data in terms of both labeling the problem (e.g., *moderate to severe obstructive component, unresponsive to bronchodilator*) and determining how each value deviates from normal.

Scenario One

The patient is an eighty-year-old black male. He has a thirty-five pack-year smoking history and worked in a dusty industrial environment for twelve years. He also has a history of pneumonia and congestive heart failure. He does not admit to a regular productive cough, but does have exertional dyspnea.

Data

Parameter	Pre-Bronchodilator			Post-Bronchodilator		
	Act.	Pred.	%Pred.	Act.	Pred.	%Pred.
FVC	1.77	3.07	58%	2.17	3.07	71%
FEV_1	1.16	2.34	49%	1.84	2.34	57%
$FEV_1\%$	65%	76%	86%	62%	76%	81%
FEF_{25-75}	0.60	3.01	23%	0.73	3.01	26%
PEFR	2.69	6.53	41%	4.11	6.53	63%
MVV	33.29	111.2	30%	45.9	111.2	41%
SVC	2.6	3.07	85%	3.2	3.07	104%
IC	1.81	1.98	92%	2.19	1.98	111%
ERV	0.79	1.09	72%	1.01	1.09	92%
FRC	4.98	3.74	133%			
RV	4.19	2.65	158%			
TLC	6.79	6.12	111%			
D_LCO	14.06	23.48	60%			

Patient effort was good. Isoetharine was given as the bronchodilator. Patient is 69 inches tall and weighs 170 lbs.

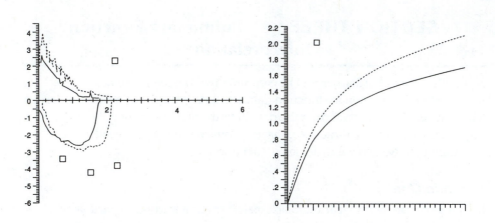

Scenario Two

The patient is a thirty-four-year-old black male with a recent history of chest pain. He has no smoking history or allergies. He denies shortness of breath; however, he has had a recent productive cough of thick yellow sputum. He is currently taking Amoxicillin.

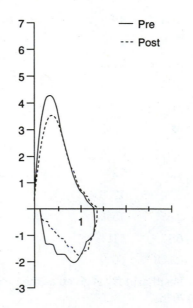

Data

Parameter	Pre-Bronchodilator			Post-Bronchodilator		
	Act.	Pred.	%Pred.	Act.	Pred.	%Pred.
FVC	1.41	5.30	27%	1.38	5.30	26%
FEV$_1$	1.22	4.35	28%	1.26	4.35	29%
FEV$_1$%	87%	82%	106%	91%	82%	111%
FEF$_{25-75}$	1.62	4.47	36%	1.89	4.47	42%
PEFR	4.40	9.49	46%	3.59	9.49	38%
SVC	1.41	5.28	26%	2.66	5.28	40%
FRC	1.69	2.73	62%	1.84	2.73	67%
RV	1.10	1.58	69%	1.25	1.58	79%
TLC	2.51	6.57	38%	2.66	6.57	40%

Scenario Three

The patient is a seventy-seven-year-old white male with a seventy-five pack-year smoking history. The patient also worked as a machinist for forty years. Recently, he has been complaining of increased shortness of breath.

Data

Parameter	Pre-Bronchodilator			Post-Bronchodilator		
	Act.	Pred.	%Pred.	Act.	Pred.	%Pred.
FVC	1.83	3.37	54%	2.27	3.37	67%
FEV$_1$	0.65	2.57	25%	0.78	2.57	30%
FEV$_1$%	35%	76%	46%	34%	76%	45%
FEF$_{25-75}$	0.23	3.41	7%	0.32	3.41	9%
PEFR	2.22	7.31	30%	3.10	7.31	42%
SVC	2.22	3.37	66%			
FRC	5.52	3.48	159%			
RV	5.08	2.46	207%			
TLC	7.30	5.69	128%			

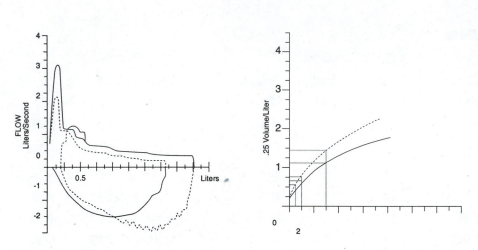

Scenario Four

The patient is a forty-six-year-old black male with a diagnosis of COPD. He has a fifteen pack-year smoking history and worked with asbestos for five years. He currently experiences frequent night sweats.

Data

	Pre-Bronchodilator			Post-Bronchodilator		
Parameter	Act.	Pred.	%Pred.	Act.	Pred.	%Pred.
FVC	5.26	5.28	100%	5.77	5.28	109%
FEV_1	3.85	4.3	89%	4.01	4.3	93%
$FEV_1\%$	73%	81%	90%	69%	81%	85%
FEF_{25-75}	140	264	53%	145	264	55%
PEFR	506	575	88%	584	575	102%
MVV	165	165	100%	177	165	107%
SVC	5.31	5.28	101%			
FRC	4.62	4.20	110%			
RV	2.18	2.27	96%			
TLC	7.49	7.35	102%			
D_LCO	27.3	26.3	104%			

Good cooperation.

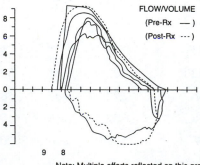

FLOW/VOLUME
(Pre-Rx ——)
(Post-Rx ---)

Note: Multiple efforts reflected on this graph.

Scenario Five

The patient is a thirty-six-year-old black female with a history of systemic lupus erythematosus. Currently, she is complaining of dyspnea and a persistent cough. She has an eighteen pack-year smoking history and no apparent occupational exposure to dust or other noxious materials. She is presently taking prednisone.

Data

Parameter	Pre-Bronchodilator			Post-Bronchodilator		
	Act.	Pred.	%Pred.	Act.	Pred.	%Pred.
FVC	1.49	3.53	42%	1.57	3.53	44%
FEV$_1$	1.16	2.77	42%	1.32	2.77	48%
FEV$_1$%	78%	78%	100%	83%	78%	106%
FEF$_{25-75}$	0.97	3.25	30%	1.44	3.25	44%
PEFR	4.25	6.20	69%	5.56	6.20	90%
SVC	1.62	3.30	49%	1.79	3.30	54%
FRC	1.92	2.61	74%			
RV	1.23	1.55	79%			
TLC	2.85	4.88	58%			

Good cooperation. Patient is 63 inches tall and weighs 150 lbs.

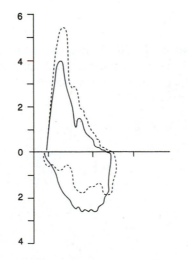

SECTION FOUR • Drug Calculations

In this section, the learner will be confronted with different clinical situations involving drug calculations. These situations are consistent with current practice.

Situation One
You are asked to administer 2 mL of 10% acetylcysteine mixed with 0.5 mL of albuterol to a patient with thick, tenacious sputum. However, the hospital pharmacy only stocks 20% acetylcysteine. How do you handle this situation?

Situation Two
You are asked to administer 250 mg of gentamicin via aerosol to a patient with bronchiectasis. The drug comes in a 4% solution. How many mL of gentamicin do you administer?

Situation Three
You are asked to administer $NaHCO_3$- to an infant in an arrest situation. The infant weighs 2.4 kg. The standard dose of $NaHCO_3$- is 2 mEq/kg of a 4.2% solution (0.5 mEq/mL). In order to administer the standard dose, how many mL of $NaHCO_3$- do you administer?

APPENDIX: RATIONALES

CHAPTER ONE • Rationale

Patient 1: Linda Loman

Apparent Cardiopulmonary Problem

The patient appears to have a left pleural effusion. This is suggested on the basis of the combination of dull percussion note and decreased vocal fremitus in the left base. The decreased chest excursion on the left side and very decreased breath sounds are also contributing factors. In addition, pleural effusion is frequently a complication of lung cancer.

Additional Useful Information

A chest x-ray would confirm the physical findings; arterial blood gases would be useful in determining level of hypoxemia and ability to ventilate adequately.

Suggested Basic Treatment

If the patient does have a pleural effusion, she will require a thoracentesis to drain the fluid; she may also require the placement of a chest tube depending on the nature of the fluid removed. In addition, she would probably benefit from oxygen.

Patient 2: Mary Malloy

Apparent Cardiopulmonary Problem

The patient appears to have a right middle lobe consolidation, probably from pneumonia. This is suggested mostly by the increased vocal fremitus and dull percussion over the right middle lobe. The fine crackles in this area are also a contributing factor. The fact that the patient has an increased temperature suggests an infection. Her overall appearance suggests a lack of proper medical care.

Additional Useful Information

A chest x-ray would confirm the physical findings. Arterial blood gases would be useful to document hypoxemia. If the patient has a productive cough, a sputum specimen might help in determining the causitive microorganism. A recent history would also be useful.

Suggested Basic Treatment

Until the microorganism is determined, a broad spectrum antibiotic might be useful. Oxygen would also be helpful. Other respiratory therapeutic modalities that promote bronchial hygiene might also be useful.

Patient 3: J.C. Pierce

Apparent Cardiopulmonary Problem

The patient appears to have pulmonary edema. This is suggested most by the presence of course crackles on inspiration throughout both lung fields. The patient does not have a significant temperature, and the vocal fremitus is not increased anywhere; therefore, pneumonia and consolidation can likely be ruled out.

Additional Useful Information

Again, a chest x-ray would confirm the physical findings. Arterial blood gases would determine the extent of the hypoxemia (suggested from the presence of cyanosis). A patient history would be useful in determining the degree of cardiac decompensation.

Suggested Basic Treatment

The patient would benefit from oxygen therapy. Appropriate drug therapy to treat the edema should be initiated by the attending physician.

Patient 4: Jake McCandles

Apparent Cardiopulmonary Problem

The patient appears to have a right side consolidation, concentrated mostly in the right base. This is suggested by the presence of dull percussion and bronchial breath sounds in this area. Since the patient is unresponsive, obviously vocal fremitus cannot be obtained. The increased temperature also suggests pneumonia (which is the admitting diagnosis).

Additional Useful Information

Again, a chest x-ray would confirm the physical findings. Arterial blood gases w·uld be useful in determining degree of hypoxemia. A recent medical history of the patient would also be useful, especially considering the age of the patient (forty-five) compared to his overall physical condition (poor). A sputum specimen would be useful in determining the causitive microorganism.

Suggested Basic Treatment

Appropriate antibiotic therapy should be initiated by the attending physician. Oxygen therapy would probably be useful. Other respiratory therapy modalities to promote bronchial hygiene might also be useful.

Patient 5: Alex Dwyer

Apparent Cardiopulmonary Problem

The patient appears to be having an asthma attack. This is suggested most by the breath sounds (wheezing superimposed over a prolonged expiratory phase).

Additional Useful Information

Arterial blood gases might be useful in determining presence of hypoxemia and in determining ability to ventilate adequately. The presence of a productive cough and the nature of the sputum would also be useful information. In addition, a patient history would be very useful: does this patient have a history of asthma or is this an isolated incident? Questioning of this sort might reveal information that would be useful in determining proper therapy.

Suggested Basic Treatment

A quick acting inhaled bronchodilator would be most useful at this point in time (or at least until additional information can be obtained). The patient would probably also benefit from oxygen therapy.

Patient 6: Katherine McClintock

Apparent Cardiopulmonary Problem

The patient appears to have a left pneumothorax. This is suggested mostly by the absence of breath sounds and the hyperresonant percussion note over the left side. Her recent automobile accident with chest trauma also contributes to the suspicion.

Additional Useful Information

A chest x-ray would confirm the physical findings. Arterial blood gases would also be useful (although this is an emergency situation).

Suggested Basic Treatment

If the patient does have a pneumothorax, a chest tube needs to be placed immediately. Oxygen therapy would probably also be beneficial.

Patient 7: Fenton Hardy

Apparent Cardiopulmonary Problem

The patient appears to have a right basilar consolidation. This is suggested by the dull percussion and fine crackles over this area. The patient's overall appearance also contributes to the diagnosis of pneumonia. The rhonchi suggest the presence of retained secretions.

Additional Useful Information

A chest x-ray would confirm the physical findings. A sputum specimen would also be useful.

Suggested Basic Treatment

Appropriate antibiotic therapy should be initiated by the attending physician. Oxygen therapy is indicated in the presence of documented hypoxemia. The presence of rhonchi suggest that bronchial hygiene might be useful.

Patient 8: Chet Morton

Apparent Cardiopulmonary Problem

The patient appears to be suffering an acute exacerbation of chronic bronchitis. All of the physical findings and lab data are typical of chronic bronchitis.

Additional Useful Information

A recent medical history would be useful in determining home therapy and onset of symptoms. A sputum specimen would be useful in determining the presence of an infection.

Suggested Basic Treatment

The patient is already on oxygen; additional oxygen therapy is open to debate. Bronchial hygiene and inhaled bronchodilators would probably be useful. The patient should be closely monitored for signs of fatigue.

Patient 9: Wilma Wagg

Apparent Cardiopulmonary Problem

The patient appears to be experiencing an acute exacerbation of emphysema. All of the patient's physical findings and lab data are classic for emphysema.

Additional Useful Information

A recent medical history would be useful. If the patient has a productive cough, a sputum specimen would also be useful.

Suggested Basic Treatment

Although the patient is already receiving oxygen, she could also benefit from an increased amount. In addition, she might benefit from bronchial hygiene and inhaled bronchodilators (although the need for such therapy is not as obvious in her case as it was with Chet Morton).

Patient 10: Trisha Foder

Apparent Cardiopulmonary Problem

The patient appears to be experiencing a severe form of reactive airway disease (RAD). This is suggested by the slightly hyperresonant percussion note and prolonged expiratory phase. The fact that wheezing is not heard does not eliminate RAD (or asthma) from consideration since air movement is obviously very limited.

Additional Useful Information

In this case, additional information is crucial in order to confirm the reactive airway episode. A chest x-ray might rule out spontaneous pneumothorax. A positive patient history of asthma or other chronic obstructive disease would suggest that is another exacerbation. The environment immediately preceding the patient's initial onset of shortness of breath would also be useful. A peak flow reading might help to confirm decreased lung function.

Suggested Basic Treatment

If this is an acute exacerbation of RAD, inhaled bronchodilators are most indicated. Peak flow readings before and after bronchodilator administration would help to monitor the effectiveness of such therapy.

CHAPTER TWO • Rationale

Patient 1: I. M. Quick

The patient is suffering from an acute exacerbation of COPD; he is also a CO_2 retainer (from the blood gases). The oxygen order of 0.28 air entrainment mask is probably the most appropriate. The patient might also benefit from an aerosolized bronchodilator and bronchial hygiene (postural drainage and percussion to patient tolerance).

Patient 2: Adolph Petroni

The patient is suffering from an exacerbation of COPD; he also appears to be a CO_2 retainer (by blood gases). Because of the risk of over oxygenation blunting the patient's hypoxic drive, the oxygen order of 6 Lpm is too high; either an air entrainment mask at 24% or 28%, or a nasal cannula at 1 to 3 Lpm would be safer. The patient might also benefit from an aerosolized bronchodilator and bronchial hygiene.

Patient 3: Mary Pusche

The patient is suffering from pneumonia superimposed over her lung cancer (a chest x-ray would be useful in establishing a diagnosis). The oxygen order of simple mask at 3 Lpm is not technically correct since simple masks should be a minimum of 5 Lpm. The patient does require a moderate amount of oxygen (e.g., nasal cannula 4 to 6 Lpm or simple mask at 5 or 6 Lpm). She might also benefit from bronchial hygiene, but caution must be taken, especially if any hemoptysis occurs during therapy. She could also use some packed red cells.

Patient 4: Philip Folkstone

This patient is suffering from acute pulmonary edema. He definitely requires oxygen, but the order of nasal cannula at 4 Lpm is too conservative for this patient. He has a significant cardiac stress situation which requires complete elimination of hypoxemia. The patient should be placed on at least 6 Lpm or a partial or nonrebreathing mask; there is no short term risk to the patient in using this much oxygen. Blood gases should be repeated soon after the change, and the patient should be monitored closely for signs of fatigue.

Patient 5: Bronco Lane

The patient is suffering an acute exacerbation of pulmonary fibrosis—a basically untreatable condition. The patient clearly needs a moderate amount of oxygen. The choice of device (nasal catheter) would certainly have to be questioned on the basis of patient comfort alone. The patient should be on at least 4 to 6 Lpm of oxygen to help eliminate the dyspnea. In addition, if the patient begins to show signs of fatigue, IPPB (or perhaps some other noninvasive ventilation) should be considered.

Patient 6: Brewster Baker

The patient is suffering from a myocardial infarction. There are no apparent pulmonary complications. Oxygen is clearly indicated to reduce cardiac stress. The simple mask at 5 Lpm is one appropriate method of oxygen delivery. A nasal cannula may be substituted if patient does not tolerate the mask.

Patient 7: Laurie Cable

The patient is apparently suffering from an acute asthma episode. The oxygen order of nasal cannula at 6 Lpm seems a little drastic for a SpO_2 of 92%, but it is probably not harmful over the short term. The patient really needs a sequence of aerosolized bronchodilator (e.g., 0.5cc albuterol in 2.5cc normal saline Q. 20 minutes x 3). In addition, her peak flow before and after therapy should be monitored.

Patient 8: Marion Ravenwood

The patient appears to be suffering from postoperative atelectasis and possibly pneumonia. Oxygen would appear to be indicated from her SpO_2 of 93% on room air. The mask is probably okay; but the patient might tolerate a nasal cannula a bit better. The patient would also benefit from some hyperinflation therapy and possibly bronchial hygiene (perhaps a combination of incentive spirometry and aerosol therapy).

Patient 9: Julio Delgado

The patient is suffering from an acute exacerbation of bronchiectasis, a disease in which a large amount of sputum is produced. The oxygen therapy order seems appropriate, although a higher liter flow would probably not be harmful. The patient really needs aerosolized bronchodilator therapy and vigorous bronchial hygiene. He might even benefit from an aerosolized mucolytic agent.

Patient 10: Wilma Dearing

The patient is suffering from an exacerbation of COPD. The patient is a CO_2 retainer by blood gases. The oxygen therapy order in this case is dangerous—her PaO_2 is already as high as it should be. Her increasing CO_2 is a source of concern—the patient should be closely monitored for signs of fatigue. She would probably benefit from an aerosolized bronchodilator and some bronchial hygiene (e.g., 0.5cc albuterol in 2.5cc normal saline Q. 4h.).

Patient 11: Gracie Kleidsdale

This patient appears to be suffering from pneumonia, perhaps secondary to dehydration and secretion retention. Given her present mental state, incentive spirometry would probably be extremely difficult to do. At this point in her disease progression she needs much more than hyperinflation. She would probably benefit from some vigorous bronchial hygiene. Likewise, with a PaO_2 of 49, she needs oxygen therapy—perhaps a nasal cannula at 3 to 5 Lpm or a simple mask at 5 Lpm.

Patient 12: Gene Crisby

The patient appears to be in a myasthenic crisis (although this cannot be confirmed without appropriate testing, i.e., the Tensilon test). His breathing is already shallow. The IPPB may be an appropriate therapy in this case, although one might want to add a bronchodilator for prophylactic purposes. The patient will have to be monitored closely for signs of increased ventilatory failure; this could be done by ABGs (arterial blood gases), incentive spirometry, or bedside pulmonary function testing. With a SpO_2 of 94%, the patient might benefit from supplemental oxygen.

Patient 13: Winnie Kirkwood

The patient is suffering an exacerbation of COPD. Because the patient is a CO_2 retainer, the increase in oxygen to 5 Lpm might be too much—an increase to 3 Lpm would probably be more appropriate. Also, although the patient would probably benefit from the bronchodilator, her present mental state makes administering Ventolin by MDI potentially ineffective. The route of delivery should be changed to aerosol. The patient might also benefit from postural drainage and percussion (to tolerance).

Patient 14: Kip Kiester

The patient appears to be suffering from postoperative atelectasis and possibly pneumonia (although more information would be needed to confirm that diagnosis). The patient would benefit from bronchial hygiene and hyperinflation.

The order as it is written probably does not go far enough. In addition, the selection of isoetharine as the bronchodilator might be questioned since it is shorter acting and not as beta$_2$ specific as albuterol. The SpO$_2$ of 94% on room air suggests that low flow oxygen might be indicated as well.

Patient 15: Jonathan Harker

Although the patient is in the hospital for an unrelated diagnosis (ulcerative colitis), he also appears to have secretion retention, probably related to his COPD. With this patient's history, an SpO$_2$ of 96% would seem more than adequate, and any increase in FiO$_2$ might be risky. Blood gases should be obtained. The aerosol therapy is probably indicated, although Q. 4h. might be too frequent for the patient's pulmonary condition (however, Q. 4h. probably would not be harmful either). The selection of isoetharine as the bronchodilator might be questioned (see Case Fourteen).

Patient 16: Mina Seward

This patient is probably suffering from pneumonia (as in the other cases more information is needed to confirm this diagnosis). The decision to intubate her is controversial at best; however, given her mental state and her obvious secretion retention, she will probably need frequent suctioning and the endotracheal tube would provide the best access. The prescribed FiO$_2$ seems basically appropriate. She will require some form of bronchial hygiene and close monitoring.

Patient 17: Adam Troy

The patient is suffering an acute exacerbation of COPD. Given the color of the sputum and the temperature, a pulmonary infection should be suspected. The orders as written are basically appropriate. Postural drainage and percussion might be of some benefit in this case although the patient is coughing effectively on his own. A mucolytic agent might also be considered.

Patient 18: Duke Lukela

The patient is suffering from an exacerbation of silicosis. The patient appears to be breathing shallowly, which is consistent with the condition. The orders as written are okay, but of questionable benefit. Some increase in oxygen is indicated—5 Lpm seems high but not risky since the patient is not a CO$_2$ retainer. If the patient does not improve, IPPB or some form of noninvasive ventilation should be considered.

Patient 19: Philip Hogan

The patient appears to be suffering from postoperative atelectasis. He may also have a pulmonary infection superimposed over the atelectasis. The oxygen is indicated with the SpO_2 of 90%. The IPPB is a bit controversial but not contraindicated in this case. The patient does need some form of hyperinflation; however, aerosol therapy combined with incentive spirometry administered more frequently (e.g., Q. 4h.) should be effective.

Patient 20: Ann Fan

This patient is suffering an exacerbation of COPD. The increase in oxygen from 1 Lpm to 3 Lpm is of questionable benefit, but does not appear to be risky. The aerosol therapy is indicated, although the addition of the mucolytic is questionable since no sputum has yet been produced. Clearly the use of IPPB in the case of any patient with COPD has to be questioned because of the risk of barotrauma.

Patient 21: Wilbur Post

The patient appears to be suffering from pulmonary edema (although more information is needed to confirm this diagnosis). The oxygen order is okay but may not be enough—a nonrebreathing mask or high FiO_2 air entrainment mask should be considered until the patient stablizes. The patient needs to be monitored very closely for signs of increased ventilatory failure (patient is already in impending ventilatory failure). The aerosol therapy is of dubious value, but would probably not be harmful.

Patient 22: Peter Valdez

The patient appears to be suffering from atelectasis over the left base, probably related to his chest wound and the drainage of fluid from that area. With a PaO_2 of 66, an increase in FiO_2 is probably indicated—50% might be too much, but is not risky. The patient needs to re-expand the left base; IPPB should accomplish this if the patient would tolerate it. Deep breathing exercises should accomplish the same thing with less risk. Any hyperinflation therapy should coincide with appropriate pain management.

Patient 23: Helena Troy

The patient appears to be suffering an acute asthma episode which is not yet under control. The peak flow is low for her age, but without a baseline, we don't know if this is significantly low for her. The increase in oxygen is of questionable benefit, but not risky. Likewise, the use of Atrovent is questionable but not harmful. An inhaled corticosteroid (e.g., Aerobid) might be of some long term benefit. A short term increase in the administration of the inhaled beta agonist would be beneficial until the patient becomes more stable. The patient's home asthma management should also be reviewed with the patient; instruction should be given as appropriate.

Patient 24 (D): Missy Kosnowski

The patient has obvious secretion retention and a probable pulmonary infection. The aerosol therapy order is indicated. Blood gases should be obtained to determine the most appropriate approach to oxygen therapy (i.e., is the patient a CO_2 retainer). The patient would probably benefit from postural drainage and percussion following the aerosol therapy. Her home management should also be reviewed and instruction should be given as appropriate. The fact that the patient is retarded might complicate the management of this patient depending on her level of cooperation. Her retardation should not change her pulmonary management.

Patient 25 (D): Judy Dooby

The patient appears to be suffering pulmonary complications secondary to her auto accident. The SpO_2 of 94% suggests that supplemental oxygen is indicated. Likewise, the patient would probably benefit from hyperinflation therapy. Thus, these orders are appropriate as written. The patient should be monitored closely for increase or decrease in pulmonary symptoms.

CHAPTER THREE • Rationale

Patient 1: Katherine Didd

The patient appears to be suffering from a right pleural effusion or hemothorax. Further testing, including chest x-ray and arterial blood gases, is needed before any therapy can be planned. Obviously, the patient is hypoxemic on a nasal cannula at 6 Lpm (based on the SpO_2 of 88%). Therefore, she needs more oxygen—a nonrebreathing mask would be the device of choice. No other respiratory treatment can be recommended until test results are available.

Patient 2: Eddie Shoebridge

The patient is experiencing an acute exacerbation of COPD. The elevated temperature and the chest x-ray suggest pneumonia. The physical findings suggest severe secretion retention. The arterial blood gases demonstrate that the patient is a CO_2 retainer. The PaO_2 of 54 is too low, even for this patient.

Therefore, oxygen therapy needs to be initiated, either by low percent air entrainment mask (24% or 28%), or low flow oxygen by nasal cannula (1 or 2 Lpm); any higher FiO_2 is risky. The patient would probably benefit from bronchodilator therapy and bronchial hygiene—most likely aerosol treatments with 0.5cc albuterol. The patient might also benefit from the addition of a nebulized mucolytic agent (e.g., acetylcysteine) and postural drainage with percussion. Once he is through the immediate crisis, he might benefit from a pulmonary rehabilitation program and smoking cessation assistance.

Patient 3: Warren Phillips

The patient is apparently suffering an acute asthma episode. As such, no other information is really needed to determine the most appropriate immediate therapy (a before and after peak flow reading would be useful). The patient would benefit most from a series of nebulized bronchodilator treatments (e.g., 0.5cc albuterol in 2.5cc normal saline Q. 20 minutes x 3). Based on the SpO_2 of 94%, the patient is oxygenating adequately on 4 Lpm via nasal cannula—any increase in FiO_2 would be of little benefit. If the patient does not clear after three aerosol treatments, IV corticosteroids (e.g., Solu-medrol) should be considered; however, no other *inhalation* drug would be useful at this time. Since the patient is a frequent visitor to the emergency department, his home asthma management program should be reviewed with him, and specific recommendations should be made for outpatient followup (see National Asthma Education Committee guidelines).

Patient 4: Latisha Jackson

The patient appears to be suffering from laryngotracheobronchitis, however, a lateral neck x-ray would need to be taken to rule out epiglottitis. If croup is confirmed, the treatment of choice is aerosolized racemic epinepherine (0.5cc in 2.5cc normal saline). The patient might also benefit from a cool mist tent with oxygen. The patient is hypoxemic on room air based on the SpO_2 of 88%. She should also be kept as quiet as possible.

Patient 5: Willie Fremont

The patient appears to be experiencing atelectasis, probably post-operative. He may also have secretion retention and quite possibly pneumonia (based on increased temperature and WBC count). He would benefit from bronchial hygiene and hyperinflation therapy—possibly aerosol therapy with postural drainage and percussion (keeping his post-operative status in mind). The patient still has moderate hypoxemia on the nasal cannula at 2 Lpm; therefore, an increase in FiO_2 would be appropriate.

Patient 6: Hans Lipper

The patient's physical findings and chest x-ray are consistent with histoplasmosis. The patient will need some form of bronchial hygiene (i.e., aerosol therapy and possibly postural drainage with percussion). The patient is also hypoxemic on room air and thus would probably benefit from low FiO_2 oxygen therapy. A sample of the sputum should be collected for cytologic examination to help confirm the diagnosis.

Patient 7: Barry Burnerd

The patient is experiencing secretion retention and possibly mild pneumonia as a result of the artificial airway in place. The patient would probably benefit from bronchial hygiene administered in the form of intermittent aerosol therapy, with a bronchodilator and possibly a mucolytic agent. Postural drainage and percussion would be beneficial but is risky due to the multiple rib fractures. The patient is not hypoxemic on 40% oxygen, therefore, increased FiO_2 would be of no benefit. A sample of the sputum would be useful for a culture and sensitivity.

Patient 8: Pogue McPherson

The patient is experiencing post-operative atelectasis and quite possibly pneumonia. This condition may be exacerbated by his obesity. Bronchial hygiene would be the treatment of choice. Postural drainage and percussion would also be indicated. However, his obesity would make this difficult to implement effectively. A chest x-ray would be useful to detect the presence of pneumonia. He is hypoxemic on room air, therefore, oxygen at low FiO_2 would also be indicated.

Patient 9: Horace Forest

The patient may have secretion retention or pneumonia superimposed over the sarcoidosis. Aerosol therapy with a bronchodilator would be indicated in this case. The patient is hypoxemic on room air, therefore, low FiO_2 oxygen therapy is also indicated. Not much else can be done to effectively deal with the underlying disease process.

Patient 10: LaWanda Harris

Apart from the pneumonia, the patient is most likely suffering an acute exacerbation of COPD. The main feature of this case is the fact that she is a CO_2 retainer and is receiving too much oxygen (40%). That accounts for her elevated $PaCO_2$ and her drowsiness (possible CO_2 narcosis). The first priority is to lower the FiO_2. The patient would also benefit from aerosol therapy with a bronchodilator as she most likely has some bronchospasm and secretion retention. Once the FiO_2 is changed, followup arterial blood gases will be necessary.

Patient 11: Mitzi Winston

The patient seems to be suffering from some sort of progressive neuromuscular disease, quite possibly Guillain-Barré syndrome (although a spinal tap would need to be done to confirm this). Nothing can be done to stop the progression. However, the patient should be monitored on a regular basis for signs of increased deterioration (e.g., hourly incentive spirometry or peak flow measurements). The PaO_2 on room air is adequate at the present time—no oxygen therapy is needed at this time.

Patient 12: Homer Folk

The patient appears to be experiencing acute pulmonary edema secondary to his congestive heart failure. Little respiratory therapy can be done that would be of any benefit in reversing the condition—the edema must be treated pharmacologically. However, the patient does need much more oxygen than 3 Lpm. A nonrebreathing mask is probably the device of choice. The patient might also benefit from mask CPAP. The patient will need to be monitored closely since he is already demonstrating signs of ventilatory fatigue (elevated $PaCO_2$), and could progress to acute ventilatory failure very quickly.

Patient 13: B. J. Stooker

The patient is experiencing an exacerbation of black lung disease. Since secretion retention is not obvious from the physical findings, bronchial hygiene might be of limited value. However the patient probably would benefit from hyperinflation therapy, most likely in the form of IPPB. The patient is hypoxemic on room air, and would benefit from low FiO_2 oxygen therapy. Nothing can be done to reverse the lung damage.

Patient 14: Jack Speck

The patient appears to be experiencing post-episode atelectasis and pneumonia (although this would need to be confirmed with a chest x-ray and a sputum culture and sensitivity). This will need to be treated with bronchial hygiene modalities. However due to the high probability of increased intracranial pressure postural drainage is risky. In addition, in case of an ineffective cough, nasotracheal suction might also raise the ICP. Oxygenation is still marginally inadequate at 6 Lpm; therefore, an increase in FiO_2 should be considered.

Patient 15: Lucy Minster

The patient appears to be experiencing pneumonia. She probably has secretion retention as well. She will need bronchial hygiene. However, because of her age and condition (arthritis, debility, etc.), she will probably not tolerate any aggressive therapy. She will need to be monitored closely for any evidence of further deterioration. Her PaO_2 is obviously inadequate at 47. Oxygen administered at low FiO_2 needs to be instituted. Pulse oximetry should be substituted for a follow up blood gas.

Patient 16: Ann Felson

The patient appears to be experiencing atelectasis over the right hemithorax. Any bronchial hygiene and/or hyperinflation therapy would be risky because of the hemoptysis since the patient may have active pulmonary bleeding. The PaO_2 at 6 Lpm is adequate; however, the patient will need to be monitored closely for evidence of further deterioration.

Patient 17: Leroy Wilson

Based on the chest x-ray, physical findings, and diagnosis, the patient appears to be experiencing a right pleural effusion. A thoracentesis will need to be done before any additional respiratory therapy procedures are recommended. The patient's PaO_2 is marginal at 4 Lpm. The liter flow could be increased.

Patient 18: James Plato

Even though the patient is admitted for gastrointestinal problems his history of bronchiectasis will require attention. Appropriate aerosol therapy and postural drainage and percussion is indicated. The patient is hypoxemic but is also a CO_2 retainer. Therefore, oxygen may not be necessary. Certainly any FiO_2 that raises the PaO_2 much above 65 would be risky. The patient will need to be monitored closely for signs of exacerbation of the bronchiectasis.

Patient 19: Wally Winters

The patient is experiencing a typical exacerbation of cystic fibrosis. Therefore, he will need to be treated with aerosol therapy and postural drainage with percussion. He is receiving appropriate oxygen therapy—any increase in FiO_2 will be risky. Prior to discharge, his home management program should be reviewed.

Patient 20: Foster Lacey

The patient has crackles in the lung bases that may be related to early pulmonary edema. Otherwise, there is no evidence of active pulmonary involvement. PaO_2 is too low for his condition, even on 3 Lpm. Therefore, the FiO_2 should be increased either to 6 Lpm or possibly to a high FiO_2 air entrainment mask. He will need to be monitored closely, perhaps with continuous pulse oximetry. The history of alcohol abuse and liver problems is not particularly relevant to respiratory care.

Patient 21: Meredith Fooster

The patient is probably experiencing significant secretion retention secondary to the pneumonia and possibly the dehydration. She will benefit from appropriate bronchial hygiene and possibly bronchodilator therapy. Secretion removal is difficult to assess in infants because they cannot expectorate. The oxygen therapy is probably adequate at the 2 Lpm flow; however, the SpO_2 should be monitored closely.

Patient 22: Mandy Mason

The patient is experiencing airway narrowing secondary to the bronchiolitis. She will benefit most from appropriate bronchodilator therapy. Her SpO_2 of 89% on room air suggests hypoxemia and should be treated, possibly with a nasal cannula at a low flow. The SpO_2 should be monitored closely.

Patient 23: Sean Wiggins

On the surface, this seems to be a relatively simple case in that the patient has secretion retention and will benefit from bronchial hygiene. However, with the diagnosis of oat-cell carcinoma, comfort measures should be a priority since the patient will in all likelihood deteriorate rapidly. Also, bronchial hygiene is potentially risky since the patient has significant hemoptysis. The PaO_2 is marginally adequate on 3 Lpm—it could be increased.

Patient 24: Willie Lawson

The patient is apparently experiencing an exacerbation of the underlying COPD, quite possibly a lung infection. Since he is at home, he needs to see his doctor as soon as possible. In addition his SpO_2 on room air is too low. He should be encouraged to use his oxygen as prescribed (at least 2 to 3 Lpm). A followup visit over the next few days is important.

Patient 25: Neil Armitron

There are two predominant features of this case: 1) the patient is overusing his beta-adrenergic inhaler, 2) his SpO_2 is very low, even on 4 Lpm. The increased inhaler use may indicate a deterioration of the condition—the addition of inhaled or maybe even systemic corticosteroids should be considered. He would also benefit from breathing retraining exercises, since the increased inhaler use might simply be related to the momentary desaturation that occurs with exertion. The decreased SpO_2 is obviously not a sudden condition since his hematocrit is so high. His liter flow should be increased; a transtracheal catheter insertion should be considered.

CHAPTER FOUR • Rationale

Patient 1: Arnie Lovelow

Arterial blood gases do not justify mechanical ventilation at this time. However, the change in condition is a problem along with the severe hypoxemia. At this point, aggressive bronchial hygiene along with an increase in oxygen should be enough to stabilize the patient. Also, the fact that the patient has COPD must be factored into the decision making process.

Patient 2: Mary Gay

This patient is in impending ventilatory failure (by arterial blood gases) in addition to being severely hypoxemic on a high FiO_2. However, appropriate medical management should cause her CHF to reverse in a few hours, thus easing her work of breathing. Because of this, she might be a candidate for noninvasive pressure support (e.g., BiPAP via nasal mask). If this does not work or if she does not tolerate the mask, she should be placed on a volume ventilator with settings appropriate to her height and weight and an FiO_2 to start. Cardiac indicators (e.g., heart rate, blood pressure, urinary output) should be monitored closely. The FiO_2 should be titrated to the SpO_2.

Patient 3: Filo Bedlam

The arterial blood gases and clinical indicators are not bad enough to justify mechanical ventilation at this time. In addition, the low blood pressure might be exacerbated by the positive pressure ventilation. He would benefit from an increase in oxygen therapy (possibly 50% to 70%) and aggressive bronchial hygiene.

Patient 4: Jennifer Yaslov

Arterial blood gases and clinical indicators suggest a need for ventilatory support. Her condition will probably continue to deteriorate. She should be placed on a volume ventilator (with low volume capability). Tidal volume should be titrated to height and weight; minute ventilation should be titrated to $PaCO_2$ levels. FiO_2 should be set to maintain an SpO_2 above 92% (increased temperature will increase oxygen consumption).

Patient 5: Forrest Grange

This patient is in clear ventilator failure and will clearly require ventilatory support in order to survive. He may be developing pneumonia. His condition and primary diagnosis suggest a poor prognosis even with aggressive therapy. Therefore, certain ethical issues must be considered before committing him to life support.

Patient 6: Anthony Angle

This patient appears to be developing ventilatory failure, perhaps secondary to cerebral bleeding. Therefore, the patient will probably require ventilatory support. The attending physicians may wish to titrate his minute volume to his intracranial pressure. The patient should be placed on a volume ventilator. The FiO_2 should be adjusted to keep the SpO_2 above 90%.

Patient 7: Pippi Longnecker

The patient is in ventilatory failure secondary to the drug overdose. Even though she is not hypoxemic, she is obviously hypoventilating. Because of the hypoventilation it is only a matter of time before the slow, shallow breathing causes atelectasis and serious ventilation/perfusion problems. Thus, she needs ventilatory support. Because of the possible transient nature of her underlying pathology, she may be managed by noninvasive means (e.g., BiPAP via nasal mask). Otherwise, if the decision is made to intubate and insitute conventional mechanical ventilation, the rate and tidal volume should be set according to her body weight; the FiO_2 doesn't need to be higher than 35%. Since she is spontaneously breathing, consideration might be given to placing her on SIMV (synchronized intermittent mandatory ventilation) to start.

Patient 8: John Stryker

This is a very borderline situation, with the patient beginning to show signs of ventilatory failure. Consideration might be given to noninvasive ventilatory support (e.g., BiPAP); however secretion management might be a problem. The patient is currently receiving aggressive bronchial hygiene. It is too early to know if this will be effective. Therapy might be increased to Q. 1h. or Q. 2h. for the next few hours with consideration given to noninvasive pressure support ventilation. However, if the decision is made to intubate and ventilate, V_E needs to be set carefully since the patient is a CO_2 retainer and the pH is not that far from normal.

Patient 9: Sybil Gordon

This patient is beginning to show signs of fatigue (increasing $PaCO_2$, severe hypoxemia on 6 Lpm of oxygen). Inhaled beta agonists are apparently not effective; peak flow is very low. However, because she will be difficult to ventilate and because Solu-medrol takes several hours to peak, consideration should be given to continuing the inhaled beta agonists and monitoring her closely for signs of further deterioration. If the decision is made to ventilate, close attention must be paid to tidal volume, plateau pressure, inspiratory time, and auto-PEEP (positive end-expiratory pressure) must be measured. If she is not paralyzed, she should probably be placed on SIMV at settings which will insure an I:E ratio of at least 1:3 or 1:4. Aerosol therapy must be continued through the ventilator.

Patient 10: Baby Girl Gomez

The patient is in obvious respiratory distress and ventilatory failure. She should be placed on a time cycled, pressure limited ventilator. Inspiratory time should be prolonged and pressure limit should be titrated to chest rise and breath sounds. FiO_2 should start at 100%; PEEP should be set at 5cm to 10cm H_2O. She will need to be monitored closely. Artificial surfactant should be given.

Patient 11: Anna Clarkstown

The patient appears to be suffering from pneumonia. Although she has severe hypoxemia, she is ventilating adequately. Because of her age, vegetative state and apparent dehydration, she is not a good candidate for mechanical ventilation. Instead, aggressive bronchial hygiene should be instituted. Oxygen should be administered by a mask that delivers medium to high FiO_2 (e.g., 50% to 60% air entrainment mask or nonrebreathing mask).

Patient 12: Tuco Ramirez

At the moment, the patient is not weak enough to require mechanical ventilation. Conventional therapy might eliminate the crisis before the patient gets much worse. The patient should be monitored closely. This could be accomplished through frequent vital capacity measurements, peak flow measurements, incentive spirometry, or arterial blood gases (for $PaCO_2$ changes).

CHAPTER FIVE • Rationale

Patient 1: Alvy Singer

This patient was admitted for viral pneumonia and developed ventilatory failure and probable severe secretion retention. Compliance is relatively low and resistance is relatively high, even after the implementation of mechanical ventilation. Because of the thickness of the sputum, the HME should be replaced with a heated humidifier. In addition, the $PaCO_2$ is low; therefore, the V_E should be decreased. Because the patient is not assisting at this time, this decrease would be best accomplished by decreasing the respiratory rate. Consideration could be given to decreasing the FiO_2, especially since the FiO_2 of 1.0 might lead to oxygen toxicity. However, conventional wisdom dictates that only one ventilator change be made at a time. The patient might also benefit from chest percussion.

Patient 2: Samantha Eastway

This patient is suffering an acute asthma episode. Airway resistance is very high, and the beta agonists do not seem to be breaking the bronchospasm. After almost twenty-four hours, the airway resistance seems to be a little better. The $PaCO_2$ is a little high but still within normal limits; therefore, the V_E doesn't need to be increased, especially considering the very real possibility of airtrapping. Auto-PEEP should be measured. In all likelihood, the patient should be maintained as is with a continuation of the frequent albuterol treatments. The patient should be monitored closely for signs of recovery.

Patient 3: Bertha Ferrentino

The patient is experiencing an acute exacerbation of her COPD. Airway resistance was high. At the present time, the patient seems to have stabilized on the ventilator; ABGs have normalized. The patient is doing more spontaneous breathing. Consideration should be given to obtaining weaning parameters and perhaps adding pressure support in order to overcome the resistance of the ET tube and facilitate decreasing the intermittent mandatory ventilation (IMV) rate in anticipation of weaning. Decreasing the FiO_2 to 30% might also serve to stimulate spontaneous ventilation since she is a CO_2 retainer.

Patient 4: Anton Garcia

This patient has developed adult respiratory distress syndrome with its attendant compliance decrease and capillary leaking problems. Now, two days later, the patient has improved very little. The hemodynamic parameters suggest some interference with cardiac function, perhaps due to high pulmonary vascular resistance. Also, the $PaCO_2$ is rising. Some thought might be given to pressure control ventilation to minimize the risk of barotrauma. Also, the patient might be better maintained at the higher $PaCO_2$ level (permissive hypercapnia). The cardiac output and the pulmonary capillary wedge pressure (PCWP) need to be monitored closely. Urinary output should also be monitored closely.

Patient 5: Samuel Peppercorn

The patient was placed on the ventilator because of ventilatory failure secondary to the surgical condition and post-operative management. The patient is now assisting and is agitated. ABGs show hyperventilation with hyperoxemia. Consideration should be given to decreasing the FiO_2, especially considering the eventual risk of oxygen toxicity. Because the patient is assisting and is agitated, consideration might also be given the putting the patient on SIMV with pressure support. The right side will have to be monitored closely, especially for signs of additional bleeding. The left side will have to be monitored for signs of volutrauma because the majority of inspired volume will be distributed to the left side as long as it is more compliant.

Patient 6: Freda Watkins

This patient had open heart surgery but did not come off the ventilator as planned. This was possibly due to her pre-existing COPD. Airway resistance was high. At present, the patient is alert and oriented. ABGs are good; the chest x-ray is fairly typical of the immediate postoperative period. Cardiac output is fair. Since the PaO_2 is 118, the FiO_2 should be decreased. In addition, since the patient is alert and assisting, consideration should also be given to obtaining weaning parameters. Placing the patient on SIMV with pressure support might stabilize the $PaCO_2$ and facilitate weaning. She might also benefit from mild chest percussion since she appears to have some secretion retention.

Patient 7: Lorita Menendez

This patient was admitted and placed on the ventilator because of ventilatory failure due to Guillain-Barré Syndrome. The disease appears to be running its course, and now the patient is beginning to show signs of recovery. She appears to have stabilized on the ventilator. Consideration might be given to decreasing the FiO_2, although this would have limited value. Consideration might also be given to obtaining weaning values. She should be monitored closely for additional signs of recovery. She also seems to be developing secretion retention with a possible infection. She might benefit from in-line aerosol therapy and chest physiotherapy.

Patient 8: Joseph Abramowitz

This is a patient who developed severe cardiopulmonary problems secondary to postoperative problems. Now he is a failure to wean from the ventilator and is in a subacute care facility. Basically, he is stable on the ventilator; however, with the increase in the thickness of the secretions and the change in color, it is apparent that an infection might be developing. He needs to be monitored closely for pneumonia. He might benefit from in-line aerosol therapy and chest percussion. Consideration might also be given to obtaining weaning parameters once the infection has cleared.

Patient 9: Nellie Wanamaker

This is a patient who apparently developed pneumonia and was transferred from a nursing home. She is a debilitated patient who probably has stabilized on the ventilator and may never be able to be weaned. Her nutritional status should be monitored closely. Consideration might also be given to gradually decreasing the IMV rate (e.g., 2 Bpm every other day) and monitoring clinical signs of ventilatory failure (e.g., increased work of breathing, increased heart rate, etc.).

Patient 10: Nolan Sanchez

This patient was placed on the ventilator in order to titrate the intracranial pressure with the $PaCO_2$. At present the chest has stabilized; however, the $PaCO_2$ is up slightly. Even though the $PaCO_2$ is normal and the pH is acceptable, the rise in $PaCO_2$ might interfere with the desired decrease in intercranial pressure (ICP). Therefore, some consideration might be given to increasing the V_E possibly by raising the rate back to 18. In addition, the metabolic acidosis needs to be monitored.

Patient 11: Baby Boy Francini

This patient has meconium aspiration with apparent loss of lung compliance. The Survanta trial appears to have been somewhat successful, although the $PaCO_2$ is still a bit high. This will need to be monitored closely, since any increase in compliance might lead to increased volume delivery with the risk of barotrauma. Consideration should be given to reducing the FiO_2 since the patient is at risk for oxygen toxicity.

Patient 12: Baby Girl Hank

This patient was born prematurely and has probably developed IRDs. However, at present, her ABGs are marginal on ventilator settings that are pushing the limits of safety. Some consideration might be given to increasing the respiratory rate since the PIP is already relatively high. The patient should be monitored closely for increased signs of failure. Consideration might also be given to alternative methods of support, such as, jet ventilation, and/or extracorporeal membrane oxygenation. Artificial surfactant should be administered as soon as possible after delivery.

CHAPTER SIX   •   Rationale

Clinical Situation 1

In this situation, you obviously cannot be in two places at the same time; therefore, you must decide which code is the higher priority. Some of your decision will be based on the other personnel available at each code and how well you know the abilities of this personnel. Emergency departments should be independently equipped to handle code situations, and most emergency department physicians are able to intubate. If this is the case, then you should remain at the ICU code until the patient is stabilized. You may request that an ancillary staff person call to the emergency department and obtain a status report on the patient there.

Clinical Situation 2

This is usually a fairly simple problem to correct. The problem is caused when the wall outlet seal does not retract. You should simply place the flowmeter back into the wall thus sealing the outlet. If this does not stop the oxygen, you can turn off the zone valve for that unit; however, by so doing, you are turning off the oxygen to all of the rooms. Obviously, under these conditions, you must provide an alternative oxygen source for those patients who need it.

Clinical Situation 3

This is another situation in which you cannot be in two places at the same time. The most logical course of action would be to see if another therapist can perform one of the procedures for you. If this is not possible, the ABGs should probably take priority over the ECG since it is more likely that therapeutic decisions will be made based on the ABG results. In addition, most physicians can do 12-lead ECGs. Under any circumstances, your decision will be based largely on a description of the two patients given to you by the requesting units. The personnel on each unit should be informed of your priorities.

Clinical Situation 4

Obviously, you cannot ignore the other patient. You should do a quick assessment of the patient to determine if the problem appears to be life threatening. Then you should inform the patient's nurse and possibly make appropriate recommendations for additional diagnostic tests (e.g., ABGs, chest x-ray) if necessary.

Clinical Situation 5

The safest course of action would be to call for help and initiate CPR, since the code status of the patient is unknown. However, this is clearly a moral dilemma.

Clinical Situation 6

Obviously, you cannot simply tell the patient what you have found. The safest answer would be to tell the patient that you have not seen any results and that the attending physician should be in sometime that day to discuss the situation with the patient.

Clinical Situation 7

This case respresents an obvious ethical and legal dilemma. First, you need to confront the legal issues associated with withdrawing life support. Next, you need to confront your own feelings about active euthenasia, which this case basically represents.

Clinical Situation 8

This is a difficult situation. You need to alert the patient (and any available family members/caregivers) to the dangers associated with smoking in the vicinity of oxygen equipment. However, you must also deal with the fact that once you leave, the patient can do whatever he wants to do. Therefore, you must thoroughly impress upon the patient not only how dangerous it is to smoke in the presence of oxygen (which may stop him from smoking with the oxygen on) but how counterproductive it is to smoke at all with his health condition. In addition, your conversation and advise to the patient should be clearly documented in the appropriate record.

Clinical Situation 9

First, the patient needs to stay calm—panic increases oxygen consumption. Second, the patient should call the electric company in order to find out when the electricity might be restored. Third, if the oxygen in the E cylinder runs out, the patient may be able to get extras from the local EMS. Fourth, if the situation gets critical, the therapist should dispatch someone from the oxygen supplier to deliver extra oxygen cylinders to the patient.

Clinical Situation 10

First, the patient needs to explore alternatives with the oxygen supplier. The insurance situation will differ from state to state. The patient may be able to take the liquid reservoir with her (assuming she has access to a vehicle that can carry it). Or she may be able to arrange to have oxygen available at her destination. The transfillable-portable should contain enough oxygen for 4 to 8 hours. She may be able to get a refill somewhere along the way, if necessary.

Clinical Situation 11

In order to accomodate the low-flow capability of concentrators and liquid reservoirs, you should probably set up a large reservoir nebulizer from an air compressor and bleed-in oxygen in order to accomplish the 35% prescription.

Clinical Situation 12

You should take the patient off the ventilator and provide ventilator support via manual resuscitator. The patient might be experiencing underlying lung problems (e.g., mucus plugging), or the ventilator itself might be malfunctioning.

CHAPTER SEVEN • Rationale

EXTENDED SITUATION 1: AMANDA ROTWILER

Part A

1. vital signs: Correct, pulse 94, BP 142/78; resp 22
2. diagnosis: Neutral, congestive heart failure
3. age: Neutral, 68
4. ABGs: Incorrect, you do not need ABG results
5. SpO_2: Correct, 96%
6. current oxygen therapy: Correct, 35% air entrainment mask
7. breath sounds: Correct, clear and decreased
8. general appearance: Correct, alert & oriented, anxious
9. pulmonary function results: Incorrect
10. chest x-ray: Neutral, some vascular enlargement, enlarged heart
11. procedure to be performed: Correct, kidney, liver scan

Part B

1. Correct, lower flow is more appropriate for transport; a mask might get in the way (number 2 is not completely incorrect since it is basically what the patient is receiving. In the real clinical simulation, this answer would take the learner to a different section of the exam which would subsequently confront the learner with a scenario that somehow forced selection of the nasal cannula at 4 Lpm; point loss for selecting this pathway would be minimal.)

Part C

2. 126 minutes

EXTENDED SITUATION 2: MOHAMMAD OMANN

Part A

4. Correct; it should be clear from the scenario that the patient is experiencing an episode of bronchospasm; while oxygen may be necessary, it will not correct the underlying problem.

Part B

1. medications taken at home: Correct, Primatene mist as needed
2. gag reflex: Incorrect
3. arterial blood gases: Correct, pH 7.51, $PaCO_2$ 24, PaO_2 60, HCO_3- 18
4. breath sounds: Correct, very decreased with slight wheezing superimposed over a prolonged expiratory phase
5. appearance of chest: Correct, normal
6. heart sounds: Incorrect, waste of time
7. methacholine challenge: Incorrect, dangerous
8. ECG: Incorrect, sinus tachycardia (a waste of time)
9. vital signs: Correct, heart rate 118, BP 146/88, Resp 26, Temp 37°C
10. sputum C&S: Incorrect, not obtained
11. history of lung disease: Correct, five emergency department visits in the last eighteen months for the same diagnosis
12. CBC: Incorrect
13. chest x-ray: Neutral, a waste of time, however showed slight hyperinflation
14. lung scan: Incorrect, dangerous
15. P_50: Incorrect
16. pulmonary function test: Incorrect, dangerous
17. peak flow: Correct, 110 Lpm
18. history of present illness: Correct, slight shortness of breath three days ago; getting progressively worse with dyspnea on exertion. Has had upper respiratory problems for the past two days

Part C

1. IV theophylline is controversial—probably would not be incorrect
5. aerosol treatments with albuterol and normal saline Q. 2h. x 4 then Q. 4h.
8. peak flow
9. oxygen via 0.50 air entrainment mask (if the PaO_2 was not that low the nasal cannula at 2 Lpm might also be acceptable but would lead the learner to a different section).

Part D

1. Place the patient on the nonrebreather mask. The learner may want to do something that is not on the list; however, this is best of the choices given.

Part E

3. Decrease the oxygen to nasal cannula at 6 Lpm; this is the best of the choices given.

Part F

2. Intal may be effective in preventing future bronchospasm from occurring.
3. Albuterol q.i.d. This is controversial since current thinking is that patients only use beta agonists on a p.r.n. basis.
5. The patient could probably benefit from an aerosolized steroid.
7. Asthma education. This patient suffers frequent relapses and is in need of some understanding of the disease process and the need for education.

EXTENDED SITUATION 3: KALYANNA SHIMATSU

Part A

4. Perform a quick assessment of the situation. You may be able to spot an obvious problem that can be corrected immediately.

Part B

1. The patient appears to be in respiratory distress.
2. Breath sounds are very decreased.
3. not taken
4. not done
5. 74 beats per minute
6. not done
7. CMV mode, rate 12, V_t 700, FiO_2 50%, flow 60 Lpm
8. 48cm H_2O
9. 642mL
10. acute exacerbation of congestive heart failure
11. ECG: sinus arrythmia with occasional PVCs
12. 74%

Part C

3. Remove the patient from the ventilator and manually ventilate. There is an obvious problem with the patient/ventilator interface. You need to trouble-shoot this problem before the patient gets any worse.

Part D

2. Lavage and suction the patient. The patient is not improving dramatically with the bagging. Thus, it appears that the problem is with the patient and not the ventilator. The fact that the patient is difficult to bag suggests some kind of obstruction, possibly a mucus plug. Lavage and suction might facilitate the removal of this plug.

Part E

2. Place the patient back on the ventilator on the original settings. It appears that the lavage and suction has corrected the problem.

EXTENDED SITUATION 4: SANFORD WILLIAMS

Part A

1. Place him on a nonrebreather mask. This is as close to 100% O_2 as it is possible to get without intubating the patient.

Part B

1. pH 7.41, $PaCO_2$ 36, HCO_3- 19, PaO_2 247
2. SpO_2 99%
3. SaO_2 59%, HbCO% 38, Hgb 14.6
4. gag reflex not done
5. breath sounds very decreased with some mild crackles in the bases
6. Heart rate 120, BP 142/68, respiratory rate 26
7. ECG not done
8. lateral neck x-rays not done
9. lung scan not done
10. portable chest shows basilar patchy infiltrates in both lungs
11. sputum culture not done
12. medical history not done
13. Patient appears to be an elderly male, minimally alert and confused, with smoke residue all over his face and some possible facial burns. Clothing appears to be smoke covered as well.

Part C

1. Intubation and mechanical ventilation. The patient clearly has carbon monoxide poisoning. The appearance of his face suggests that he may have breathed a significant amount of hot smoke and possibly sustained some inhalation burns; this puts him at high risk for developing pneumonia and ARDS. His respiratory rate and pattern make him a poor candidate for CPAP at this time.

EXTENDED SITUATION 5: JAMAL PHELPS

Part A

1. Oxygen is too cumbersome to take into the field; the symptoms described do not suggest any profound hypoxemia.
2. A Ventolin inhaler would be a good idea.
3. Intal is an inappropriate drug during an exacerbation.
4. Azmacort is not a good drug to use during an exacerbation.
5. A pulse oximeter is not necessary.
6. A portable aerosol machine and albuterol solution would be a good backup if the Ventolin by inhaler is ineffective or if Jamal has trouble with inhaler technique.
7. A stethoscope would be a good assessment tool.
8. A sphygmomanometer is not necessary.
9. The symptoms described do not suggest the need for injectable epinepherine. If his symptoms worsen enough to warrant epinepherine, he should be transported to the clinic for close observation.
10. Peak flowmeters are small and easily carried; although its value is somewhat limited in the field, a peak flow reading might be useful.

Part B

1. He has scattered expiratory wheezes superimposed over a prolonged expiratory phase.
2. He is resting comfortably with visible respirations and some mild nasal flaring.
3. Skin color is normal.
4. Capillary refill is not assessed.
5. Pupillary reaction is not assessed.

6. SpO_2 is not assessed.
7. Blood pressure is not assessed.
8. Heart rate is 106 beats per minute.
9. Respiratory rate is 26 breaths per minute.
10. Peak flow is 175 Lpm.

Part C

1. Administer 2 puffs of Ventolin via MDI and observe is the most correct response. Jamal is showing signs of an exacerbation and does need an inhaled broncho-dilator. However, he seems to be tolerating the exacerbation well enough not to transport him from the play area. He should clear in a few minutes.

Part D

1. He is anxious and in obvious respiratory discomfort.
2. Breath sounds are decreased with scattered wheezes superimposed over a prolonged expiratory phase.
3. Blood pressure is not assessed.
4. SpO_2 is 95% (although is not really necessary to assess this).
5. Peak flow is 110 Lpm.
6. Heart rate is 116 beats per minute.
7. Respiratory rate is 32 breaths per minute.
8. Skin color is normal.
9. Capillary refill time is not assessed.
10. Temperature is not taken. It is time consuming and unnecessary.

Part E

1. Theo-Dur is not recommended for use during an exacerbation.
2. Prednisone is a good idea since this is his second exacerbation of the day; he is very likely developing significant airway inflammation.
3. Epinepherine is a drug of last resort.
4. Ventolin (albuterol) times three by small volume nebulizer is the standard treatment for an exacerbation of this nature.
5. Intal is only used as a prophylactic drug.
6. EMS is not necessary.
7. Oxygen is not necessary.

EXTENDED SITUATION 6: MAYA INUNU

Part A

1. You need a collection syringe with heparin.
2. You do not need a waste syringe for an arterial puncture.
3. This would be appropriate.
4. You do not need a bigger needle unless you think you might have to perform a femoral puncture.
5. Some institutions require that puncture sites be swabbed with Betadine.
6. Sterile gauze is needed to hold pressure on the site after vena puncture.
7. Bandages may be useful; however, they should not be used as a substitute for holding pressure on the site.
8. Needle cutters are no longer used; needles must be placed in specially designated sharps containers.
9. Gloves are required.
10. A gown is optional unless the patient is in a form of isolation that requires gowns.
11. A mask is optional unless the patient is in a form of isolation that requires masks.
12. Alcohol prep pads are required to cleanse the puncture site.

Part B

1. The name is required for accurate record keeping and reporting.
2. Body temperature is not very important but can be useful for doing blood gas temperature correction during analysis.
3. Diagnosis is not that important at this stage.
4. PT and PTT would be useful to determine her ability to clot.
5. Medical history is not important at this stage.
6. Three Lpm via nasal cannula; oxygen use and device is critical to the interpretation of the oxygen parameters.
7. Medication currently being taken is not important at this stage.
8. Previous arterial blood gas results would be very useful for comparison.
9. Electrolytes might be useful if there is a metabolic problem.
10. Hemoglobin would be useful in determining oxygen availability.

Part C

4. Report the results to the patient's nurse. The results are not bad enough to require immediate action; on the other hand, they are abnormal and should be verbally reported to the patient's primary caregiver, along with recommendations appropriate to the situation if possible.

Part D

4. Perform your own assessment. The order is inappropriate. The patient is a CO_2 retainer and should probably have the oxygen lowered. However, in order to confirm this, you should perform an assessment of the patient.

Part E

1. General appearance: the patient appears to be slightly short of breath and her breathing is shallow.
2. SpO_2 is 94%.
3. Breath sounds are very decreased bilaterally.
4. Peak flow would provide little information about her ability to oxygenate.
5. The patient is oriented but seems a bit drowsy.
6. The patient is not coughing.
7. Heart rate is 88 beats per minute.
8. Respiratory rate is 26 breaths per minute.
9. Chest expansion is equal bilaterally, but decreased, especially in the bases.
10. Chest x-ray is not obtained.

Part F

4. Recommend changing to a 28% air entrainment mask. The patient is receiving too much oxygen to allow for hypoxic breathing; she needs to have the FiO_2 lowered and controlled.

EXTENDED SITUATION 7: MAIME MAST

Part A

1. Blood pressure is 110/60; not a crucial parameter.
2. Temperature is not taken.
3. Patient is alert and oriented.

4. Patient appears to be weak and cachectic.

5. Peak flow is not obtained.

6. Breath sounds are diminished throughout with crackles on inspiration.

7. No peripheral edema is noted.

8. Heart rate is 102 beats per minute.

9. The patient has a loose, nonproductive cough.

10. SpO$_2$ is 92% on a nasal cannula at 2 Lpm.

11. Chest expansion is equal bilaterally and breath sounds are decreased in the bases.

12. Respiratory rate is 24 breaths per minute.

13. The patient is predominately nonambulatory, sleeps much of the time.

14. Current medications include:

    Lasix

    Lanoxin

    Theo-Dur

    Ativan

    Atrovent (MDI)

    Compliance appears to be good, although her inhaler technique is poor.

Part B

1. Is not necessary and is expensive.

2. Is not necessary and is expensive.

3. Is not necessary and is dangerous.

4. She does not really need an oxygen increase—92% is close to normal for her age.

5. The Pulmoaide would be useful—she appears to have some secretion production that the nebulizer might help with. In addition, since her inhaler technique is poor, the nebulizer would result in better inhaled medication compliance.

6. Oral suction is worth considering—it is relatively safe and might help her expectorate.

7. There is no real indication for an inhaled steroid.

8. She is certainly not bad enough to justify a hospital admission.

Part C

1. Cleaning procedures would be good to teach.

2. No

3. Yes
4. Yes
5. Yes, oral suctioning technique only (with a Yankauer).
6. No

Part D

1. SpO_2 is 80% on the 2 Lpm from the concentrator.
2. Temperature was not obtained.
3. The patient is very sleepy.
4. The patient has been basically nonambulatory, but until yesterday was interacting well with family members.
5. The concentrator FiO_2 is 40%.
6. The Pulmoaide is working.
7. The suction machine is working—it is not necessary to check its function.
8. Blood pressure was not obtained.
9. Breath sounds are decreased throughout.
10. The sputum suctioned from the mouth is white and not too thick.

Part E

1. A new concentrator should be obtained as soon as possible.

CHAPTER EIGHT • Rationale

Section One

Scenario One

1. The arterial blood gas can be interpreted as normal acid-base state with over corrected hypoxemia.
2. Hemoblobin is very low; glucose is very low; K^+ is low, Na^+ and Cl^- are normal.
3. a. anion gap $= Na^+ - (Cl^- + HCO_3^-)$
      $142 - (97 + 24) = + 21$ mEq (high)
   b. $P(A-a)O_2 = \{[(P_B - 47) \times FiO_2] - (PaCO_2/0.8\} - PaO_2$
      $\{[(740 - 47) \times 0.80] - (38/0.8)\} - 107 = 399.9$ mm Hg (very high)
   c. $CaO_2 = (0.003 \times PaO_2) + (1.34 \times Hgb \times SaO_2)$
      $(0.003 \times 107) + (1.34 \times 6.9 \times 0.96) = 9.19$ vol% (very low)

d. $C(a-v)O_2 = CaO_2 - CvO_2$

$9.19 - [(0.003 \times 30) + (1.34 \times 6.9 \times 0.58)] = 3.7$ vol% (normal)

e. $V_D/V_T = PaCO_2 - P_ECO_2/PaCO_2$

$(38 - 32)/38 = 0.16$ (low)

f. $Q_S/Q_T = (CcO_2 - CaO_2)/(CcO_2 - CvO_2)$

$[CcO_2 = (0.003 \times P_AO_2) + (1.34 \times 6.9 \times 1.00)] = 10.76$

$(10.76 - 9.19)/(10.76 - 5.4) = 0.29$ or 29% (very high)

Scenario Two
(Note: See *Scenario One* for generic form of the equations)

1. The arterial blood gas can be interpreted as uncompensated respiratory alkalosis with over corrected hypoxemia.

2. Hemoglobin is low; Cl^- is high, K^+ and Na^+ are normal.

3. a. anion gap = $143 - (110 + 23) = 10$ mEq (low normal)

   b. $P(A-a)O_2 = \{[(750 - 47) \times 0.40] - (21/0.8)\} - 109 = 254.9$ mm Hg (very high)

   c. $CaO_2 = (0.003 \times 109) + (1.34 \times 9.2 \times 0.95) = 12.03$ vol%

Scenario Three
(Note: See *Scenario One* for generic form of the equations)

1. The arterial blood gas can be interpreted as uncompensated (or perhaps partially compensated) metabolic alkalosis with corrected hypoxemia.

2. Hemoglobin is very low; electrolytes are within normal limits.

3. a. anion gap = $138 - (95 + 34) = 9$ (low)

   b. $P(A-a)O_2 = \{[(745 - 47) \times 0.50] - (46/0.8)\} - 82 = 209.5$ mm Hg (very high)

   c. $CaO_2 = (0.003 \times 82) + (1.34 \times 7.9 \times 0.94) = 10.2$ vol%

   d. $C(a-v)O_2 = 10.2 - 6.8 = 3.4$ vol% (normal)

   e. $V_D/V_T = (46 - 36)/46 = 0.22$ (normal)

   f. $Q_S/Q_T = (11.3 - 10.2)/(11.3 - 6.9) = 0.25$ or 25% (very high)

   If $C_vO_2 = 6.77$ or 6.8

   $Q_S/Q_T = (11.3 - 10.2)/(11.3 - 6.8) = 0.24$ or 24%

Scenario Four
(Note: See *Scenario One* for generic form of the equations)

1. The arterial blood gas can be interpreted as compensated respiratory acidosis with mild uncorrected hypoxemia.

2. Hemoglobin is slightly low, but not surprising for this patient, electrolytes are normal.

3. a. anion gap = 142 – (101 + 31) = 10 mEq (low normal)

    b. $P(A\text{-}a)O_2$ = {[(735 – 47) x 0.35] – (48/0.8)} – 78 = 102.8 mm Hg (high)

    c. CaO_2 = (0.003 x 78) + (1.34 x 11.7 x 0.90) = 14.3 vol% (low)

Scenario Five

(Note: See *Scenario One* for generic form of the equations)

1. The arterial blood gas can be interpreted as uncompensated metabolic acidosis with hyperoxemia.

2. Hemoglobin is low; Na^+ and Cl^- are high, K^+ is normal

3. a. anion gap = 148 – (119 + 18) = 11 mEq (low normal)

    b. $P(A\text{-}a)O_2$ = {[(750 – 47) x 0.50] – (35/0.8)} – 24 = 83.7 mm Hg (high)

    c. CaO_2 = (0.003 x 24) + (1.34 x 9.5 x 0.96) = 12.9 vol% (low)

Scenario Six

(Note: See *Scenario One* for generic form of the equations)

1. The arterial blood gas can be interpreted as basically normal (slight respiratory alkalosis but pH within normal limits) with over corrected hypoxemia.

2. Hemoglobin is normal; K^+ is slightly low, Cl^- is high, Na^+ is normal

3. a. anion gap = 139 – (109 + 23) = 7 mEq (low)

    b. $P(A\text{-}a)O_2$ = {[(734 – 47) x 0.50] – (33/0.8)} – 141 = 161.3 mm Hg (high)

    c. CaO_2 = (0.003 x 141) + (1.34 x 13.7 x 0.97) = 18.2 vol% (normal)

    d. $C(a\text{-}v)O_2$ = 18.2 – 11.8 = 6.4 vol% (high)

    e. V_D/V_T = (33 – 20)/33 = 0.39 (normal)

    f. Q_S/Q_T = (19.3 – 18.2)/(19.3 – 11.8) = 0.15 or 15% (high)

Section Two

Scenario One

1. The arterial blood gas shows uncompensated respiratory alkalosis with over corrected hypoxemia. The systolic portion of the systemic arterial blood pressure is high, the pulmonary arterial blood pressure is high. The heart rate, cardiac output, pulmonary capillary wedge pressure, and central venous pressure are all within normal limits. The hemoglobin is slightly low for a male.

2. a. stroke volume = cardiac output (CO)/heart rate (HR)

    SV = 4.9/88 = .0557 Lpm or 55.7 mL/min (normal)

    b. cardiac index = CO/body surface area (BSA)

    (Note: BSA is obtained from the DuBois body surface area chart)

    Cl^- = 4.9/2.02 = 2.4 L (slightly low)

c. left ventricular stroke work = (SBP (systolic) − PCWP) x SV x 0.0136

    LVSW = (156 − 10) x 10 x 0.0136 = 110.6 g•m/beat (normal)

d. right ventricular stroke work = (PAP (systolic) − CVP) x SV x 0.0136

    RVSW = (36 − 5) x 55.7 x 0.0136 = 23 g•m/beat (normal)

e. systemic vascular resistance = (mean arterial pressure − CVP) x (80/CO)

    {mean arterial presure = [systolic + (2 x diastolic)]/3}

    SVR = (86 − 5) x 80/4.9 = 1241 dyne•sec/cm^5 (normal)

f. pulmonary vascular resistance = (MPAP − PCWP) x (80/CO)

    {mean pulmonary artery pressure = [PAP − systolic + (2 x diastolic)]/3}

    PVR = (25 − 10) x 80/4.9 = 245 dyne•sec/cm^5 (high)

g. static compliance = (tidal volume)/($P_{plateau}$ − PEEP)

    C_{st} = 0.6/(16 − 0) = 37.5 mL/cm H_2O (low)

h. airway resistance = (P_{peak} − $P_{plateau}$)/flow (in L/sec)

    R_{aw} = (25 − 16)/1 = 9 cm H_2O/L/sec (high)

Scenario Two

1. The arterial blood gas can be interpreted as partially compensated respiratory alkalosis with grossly over corrected hypoxema. The systemic arterial blood pressure is high, the pulmonary arterial blood pressure is high; the heart rate, pulmonary capillary wedge pressure, central venous pressure, and cardiac output are all within normal limits. The hemoglobin is low.

2. (Note: See *Scenario One* for the generic form of the equations)

   a. stroke volume = 4.7/95 = 0.0495 L or 49.5 mL (normal)

   b. cardiac index = 4.7/2.1 = 2.2 Lpm (slightly low)

   c. left ventricular stroke work = (159 − 12) x 49.5 x 0.0136 = 98.9 gm•m/beat (normal)

   d. right ventricular stroke work = (34 − 7) x 49.5 x 0.0136 = 18.2 gm•m/beat (normal)

   e. systemic vascular resistance = (105.6 − 7) x (80/4.7) = 1678.3 dyne•sec/cm^5 (high)

   f. pulmonary vascular resistance = (19.3 − 12) x (80/4.7) = 124.3 dyne•sec/cm^5 (normal)

   g. static compliance = 0.8/(19 − 0) = 0.0421 L/cm H_2O or 42.1 mL/cm H_2O (low)

   h. airway resistance = (28 − 19)/1.17 = 7.7 cm H_2O/L/sec

   i. oxygen delivery = CO x (CaO_2 x 10)

     DO_2 = 4.7 x (15.4 x 10) = 723.8 mL/min (low)

    j. oxygen comsumption $= CO \times (C_{(a-v)}O_2 \times 10)$
        $VO_2 = 4.7 \times (6.7 \times 10) = 314.9$ mL/min (high)

Scenario Three

1. The arterial blood gas can be interpreted as normal (pH is slightly below normal, but the $PaCO_2$ and the HCO_3^- are within normal limits) with mild uncorrected hypoxemia. The systemic arterial blood pressure is low while the CVP and PAP are high; the heart rate is very high. The PCWP is high; the Q_T is normal. The hemoglobin is low.

2. (Note: See *Scenario One* and *Scenario Two* for the generic form of the equations)
   a. SV $= 4/127 = 31.5$ mL (low)
   b. CI⁻ $= 4.0/1.7 = 2.4$ Lpm
   c. LVSW $= (88 - 15) \times 31.5 \times 0.0136 = 31.3$ gm•m/beat (low)
   d. RVSW $= (50 - 20) \times 31.5 \times 0.0136 = 12.9$ gm•m/beat (slightly high)
   e. SVR $= (64.7 - 20) \times (80/4) = 894$ dyne•sec/cm⁵ (normal)
   f. PVR $= (38 - 15) \times (80/4) = 460$ dyne•sec/cm⁵ (very high)
   g. $C_{st} = 1000(24 - 5) = 52.6$ mL/cm H_2O (low)
   h. $R_{aw} = 6/.83 = 7.2$ cm H_2O/L/sec (slightly high)
   i. $DO_2 = 4.0 \times (10.0 \times 10) = 400$ mL/min (low)
   j. $VO_2 = 4.0 \times (6.3 \times 10) = 252$ mL/min (normal)

Scenario Four

1. The arterial blood gas can be interpreted as uncompensated respiratory alkalosis with over corrected hypoxemia. The PAP, PCWP, and CVP are all high; the SABP, HR, and Q_T are all within normal limits. The hemoglobin is within normal limits.

2. (Note: See *Scenario One* and *Scenario Two* for the generic form of the equations)
   a. SV $= 5.7/70 = 81.4$ mL (slightly)
   b. CI⁻ $= 5.7/1.46 = 3.9$ Lpm (slightly high)
   c. LVSW $= (101 - 18) \times 81.4 \times 0.0136 = 91.9$ gm•m/beat (high)
   d. RVSW $= (67 - 17) \times 81.4 \times 0.0136 = 55.4$ gm•m/beat (high)
   e. SVR $= (65.9 - 17) \times (80/5.7) = 683.5$ dyne•sec/cm⁵ (low)
   f. PVR $= (39 - 18) \times (80/5.7) = 294.7$ dyne•sec/cm⁵ (high)
   g. $C_{st} = 800/45 = 17.8$ mL/cm H_2O (very low)
   h. $R_{aw} = 10/1 = 10$ cm H_2O/L/sec (high)
   i. $DO_2 = 5.7 \times (20.1 \times 10) = 1145.7$ mL/min (normal)
   j. $VO_2 = 5.7 \times (5.9 \times 10) = 336$ mL/min (high)

Section Three

(Note: For the purposes of interpretation, any value above 75% of what has been predicted for the patient is considered within normal limits; therefore, each value will not be listed separately as being within or outside of normal limits. Rather, an overall interpretation will be given based on the *pattern* presented by the data as a body.)

Scenario One

Moderate to severe obstructive pattern (all flows decreased, FRC and RV above normal) FVC responsive to bronchodilator, but not the FEF_{25-75} or FEV_1%; the 54% increase in PEFR may be attributable to improved effort. Diffusing capacity is decreased. No restrictive is pattern noted.

Scenario Two

Severe mixed restrictive and obstructive pattern (all volumes and flows decreased), unresponsive to bronchodilator.

Scenario Three

Severe obstructive pattern (all flows decreased, FRC, RV increased), unresponsive to bronchodilator. No restrictive pattern noted.

Scenario Four

Mild obstructive pattern (FEF_{25-75} decreased), unresponsive to bronchodilator.

Scenario Five

Severe restrictive pattern with a mild obstructive component (all volumes decreased, FEF_{25-75} decreased), FEF_{25-75} did not respond to bronchodilator, PEFR did respond suggesting possible reversal of large airway obstruction

Section Four

Situation One

Essentially, you will need to mix acetylcysteine with sterile water. The formula for determining the proper mixure is:

$V_1C_1 = V_2C_2$

$V_1 = 2$ mL

$C_1 = 10$%

$V_1 = X$

$C_2 = 20$%

$(2 \times 10) = (X \times 20) = 1$ mL

Thus, add 1 mL of sterile water to 1 mL of 20% acetylcysteine

Situation Two

In order to administer 250 mg of gentamicin, you need to determine how many mg of gentamicin there are per mL of solution. The drug comes in a 4% solution. You need to convert % to a ratio; this is done by dividing 1 by 0.04.

$1:25 = 1$ gm (solute):25 gm (solution)

1000 mg/25 mL water (1 mL of water weighs 1 gm)

40 mg/1 mL

$250/40 = 6.25$ of 4% gentamicin

Another method

$$4\% \quad = \quad 4\ g/100\ mL$$
$$= \quad 4{,}000\ mg/100\ mL$$
$$= \quad 40\ mg/mL$$
$$\text{Volume needed} \quad = \quad \frac{250\ mg}{40\ mg/mL}$$
$$= \quad 6.25\ mL$$

Situation Three

First, you need to determine how many mEq of $NaHCO_3^-$ is appropriate for the baby's weight. This is calculated by: 2 (mEq/kg) x 2.4 kg = 4.8 mEq

Next you need to determine how many mL to draw up. This is calculated by looking at the 4.2% solution being 0.5 mEq/mL: 4.8 mEq/0.5 = 9.6 mL.

You need to administer 9.6 mL of $NaHCO_3^-$. HCO_3^- must be diluted before giving it to a neonate to prevent intracranial hemorrhage due to an osmosis effect.

REFERENCES

American Association for Respiratory Care. *Aerosol Consensus Conference*. Dallas, 1991.

American Association for Respiratory Care. *Proceedings of the Second National Consensus Conference on Respiratory Care Education*. Dallas, 1993.

American College of Chest Physicians. *Mechanical Ventilation Consensus Conference*. 1993.

American Heart Association. *Textbook of Neonatal Resuscitation*. 1990.

Bills, G. W. & Soderberg, R. C. *Principles of Pharmacology for Respiratory Care*. Albany, 1994; Delmar.

Chang, D. *Respiratory Care Calculations*. Albany, 1994; Delmar.

DesJardins, T. *Cardiopulmonary Anatomy and Physiology*. Albany, 1993; Delmar.

Farzan, S. *A Concise Handbook of Respiratory Disease*. E. Norwalk, CT, 1992; Appleton & Lang.

Griffith, H. W. & Dambro, M. *The 5 Minute Clinical Consult*. Philadelphia, 1993. Lea & Febiger.

Madama, V. *Pulmonary Function Testing*. Albany, 1993; Delmar.

Mishoe, S. C. Critical thinking, educational preparation, and development of respiratory care practitioners. *Distinguished Papers Monograph*, (vol. 2, no. 1); American Association for Respiratory Care, 1993.

National Asthma Education Program. *Guidelines for the Diagnosis and Management of Asthma*. Washington, DC, 1991; National Institutes of Health.

Persing, G. *Advanced Practitioner Respiratory Care Review*. Philadelphia, 1994; Saunders.

Pilbeam, S. *Mechanical Ventilation: Physiological and Clinical Applications* (2nd ed.), Saint Louis, 1992; Mosby-Year Book.

Shapiro, B., Peruzzi, W. & Templin, R. *Clinical Application of Blood Gases* (5th ed.), Saint Louis, 1994; Mosby-Year Book.

Sills, J. *Respiratory Care Registry Guide*. Saint Louis, 1995; Mosby-Year Book.

Whitaker, K. *Comprehensive Perinatal and Pediatric Respiratory Care*. Albany, 1992; Delmar.

Wilkins, R., Krider, S. J., & Sheldon, R. *Clinical Assessment in Respiratory Care* (3rd ed.), Saint Louis, 1995; Mosby-Year Book.